Ketogenic Diet for Beginner 97 Recipes

Your Guide to High Fat, Low-Carb for Ketogenic Diet Beginners

Table Of Contents

Introduction

I think it is safe to assume that since you are reading this, you are looking for a brief handbook into the fantastic world of Ketogenic Diet! We, you have come to the right place!

Now believe me when I say that I fully understand that losing weight and keeping it under control is one of the most significant concerns of modern-day human beings. Probably you are here because of the same reason as well!

You may have already tried hundreds of different diets floating out there to no avail and are entirely disappointed right now!

 Well, the Ketogenic Diet is here to change that!

Unlike most other diets that solely focus on ultimately trimming down your calorie intake, the Ketogenic Diet takes an entirely different path and tries to restrict your carbohydrates intake.

That means you will have to forgo foods that are high in carb such as flour, sweets, cereals, potatoes, processed foods and so on.

If you do things right, then you will notice a significant reduction in your weight!

This happens because, when you start cutting down carbohydrates from your body, your body slowly enters into a state of Ketosis that turns your body into a fat burning machine!

Since I have written this bookkeeping the mindset of novices in mind, I have tried my very best to keep this book as simple and easy understand as possible.

The first two chapters of the book focus on explaining the fundamental concepts of the diet, while the remaining focus on giving you a fantastic array of heartfelt recipes for you to explore.

Chapter 1: The Fundamentals of Ketogenic Diet

Defining the Ketogenic Diet

So, let's start with the first and foremost question first.

Well, we all know that our body continually requires energy for carrying out its day to day activities right? Well, when considering the "Source" of energy, the body usually looks at carbohydrates, proteins or fat.

Unfortunately though, exposing ourselves for a long time to an high-carb – low –fat food regime have increasingly influenced our body to become dependent on glucose (coming from carbohydrates) as the primary source of energy.

Therefore, as long as we have glucose in our body, the body will always keep opting for it as the primary source of energy. The only way to deal with this is to deplete the supply of glucose so that your body is forced to look for other sources.

What does that mean? Well, if you cut down your carbohydrate intake, your body will turn to use fat as its source of energy, and start burning fat at an accelerated pace by entering Ketosis.

Therefore, the main of the Ketogenic Diet is to substantially lower down your carb intake and push your body to burn fat as the primary energy source to turn your body into a fat burning machine!

This diet is packed with a plethora of benefits that are discussed in a later chapter, but to give you an idea:

- It will help you control your appetite
- It will improve your mental clarity
- It will lower down inflammation in your body
- It will improve the stability of your blood sugar levels
- It will eliminate the risk of heartburn
- It forces your body to burn fat as energy instead of carbs
- And most importantly, it does wonders for weight loss

And just in case you are wondering, a Ketogenic Diet consists of meals that are very carefully designed to be low on the carb with moderate levels of proteins and high fat.

The next part that you should know about the diet is "Ketosis."

Understanding Ketosis

So, when you expose your body to a high-carb diet, you are always putting your body into a state of metabolic glycolysis where your body tries to get all of its energy from blood glucose.

In this state, your body experiences a spike in blood glucose after every meal that causes high levels of insulin to be released into the bloodstream. This causes your body to more fat and blocks the release of fats from fat storage.

However, when you restrict your body to a Keto friendly low-carb and high-fat diet, your body eventually goes into a state of Ketosis.

While on Ketosis, your body starts to break down fat into "Ketone Bodies" or "Ketones" that encourages your body to use Ketones as the primary source of energy.

While your body is on Ketosis, your body will start to burn fat for the energy required for day to day activities.

Whenever you are on low carbs for a few days, your body will start to adjust itself to the new form of diet and naturally kick-into ketosis.

Most cells in your body will start to use ketones and glucose for fuel and for the cells that can only take glucose, such as the parts of brain, glycerol derived from dietary fats is made into glucose by the liver through glucogenesis, which is then used by the brain.

The primary goal of the Keto Diet is to keep you in nutritional ketosis as much as possible. However, you should keep in mind that the time required for a human body to enter Ketosis varies from person to person. It might take about 4-8 weeks for your body to adjust to Ketosis fully.

However, once your body finally enters Ketosis, your glycogen level will decrease, and you will carry less water weight. Muscle endurance will increase, and you feel more energetic throughout the day.

And not to mention:

- It will help you control your appetite
- It will improve your mental clarity
- It will lower down inflammation in your body

- It will improve the stability of your blood sugar levels
- It will eliminate the risk of heartburn
- It forces your body to burn fat as energy instead of carbs
- And most importantly, it does wonders for weight loss

Regarding ketones

You may have noticed that in the previous section I have touched upon a little bit on "Ketones." Let me focus on Ketones a bit now.

A brief workflow of Ketones is as follows:

- When you deprive your body of glucose, the glycogen levels slowly deplete alongside blood sugar and insulin levels. This forces the body to look for alternative fuel sources, which in our case, is Fat.
- This is the primary effect of Ketosis!
- Once your body starts to break down fats for energy, a process known as beta-oxidation takes place, which results in the formation of Ketones that are used as fuel for brain and body.

The different types of Ketone bodies include:

- Acetone
- Acetoacetate
- Beta-hydroxybutyric acid

Understanding how your body is at Ketosis

Once you start on your Ketogenic journey, one of the first thing that you should learn is to understand how you can detect when your body is in a state of Ketosis or not.

There are many ways of doing this, but the following are the most straightforward methods that you can follow:

- Perhaps the most obvious test to follow is the breath test, where you check your breath of "Keto Breath." If you are in Ketosis, you will notice that your breath has a sort of fruity/sour or metallic feel to it. This happens due to the presence of ketone bodies such as acetone and acetoacetate.

- Another way of detecting Ketones is the urine test using urine strips. They are pretty cheap and easy to find and lets you know the level of ketones in your body with ease. Usually, a pack of 100 strips cost 10$ online.

- The most accurate one, however, is a form of a blood test known as "Blood Ketone Meter." This test is slightly expensive than the rest as the meter can cost you up to 40$ with each strip costing 5$. However, this will give you extremely accurate results. A reading between 0.5 mm to 5.0m is best for this.

Setting up a Keto pantry

Knowing what to eat and what not to eat on a Ketogenic diet is extremely crucial if you wanted to stick to nutritional ketosis. The following section will help you to prepare your pantry accordingly.

Right off the bat, processed foods and grains, including chocolates, candy, sugary drinks, pasta, bread are to be avoided.

Meats And Animal Produce: While choosing your meat, always make sure to avoid farmed animal meats and processed meats such as sausages or hot dogs.

Try to go for the animal meats and animal-derived products:

- Offal from grass-fed animals: kidney, liver, tripe, tongue, etc
- Butter
- Gelatin
- Ghee
- Pastured eggs
- Pastured poultry and pork
- Seafood caught in the wild such as caviar, crab, mussels, clams, and scallops
- Wild caught fish such as cod, mackerel, tuna, eel, etc.
- Grass-fed meat such as lamb, venison, beef, lamb, chicken, rabbit, etc.

Fats: Try to take more saturated and Monosaturated varieties of fat.

- Saturated fats include lard, tallow, duck fat, chicken fat, ghee, etc.

- Monounsaturated fats include avocado oil, olive oil, and macadamia oil
- Fats rich in poly-saturated Omega-3s extracted from animal sources
- Cocoa butter, coconut butter
- 90% or higher dark chocolate
- Palm shortening
- Chia seeds

Vegetables: When choosing your vegetable, try to avoid root vegetables and stick to the green leafy ones as they will help you to keep your carbohydrates level at a minimum.

- Watercress
- Zucchini
- Spinach
- Tomatoes
- Shallots
- Seaweeds
- Pumpkin
- Scallions
- Radishes
- Okra
- Onions
- Mushrooms
- All leafy greens
- Lettuce
- Garlic
- Fennel
- Cucumber
- Chives
- Cauliflower
- Chives
- Celery
- Carrots
- Cabbage
- Broccoli
- Bell Pepper
- Asparagus
- Artichokes

Fruits: Regarding a Ketogenic diet, most fruits are off the table, mainly because of the high level of fructose. However, small amounts of berries are allowed.

Good choices for fruits are:

- Avocado
- Olives
- Blackberry
- Lime
- Lemon
- Blueberry
- Raspberry
- Strawberry
- Cranberry

Legumes: Similar to fruits, all types of legumes are off the table. However, a minimal amount of peas or green beans can be included in your diet.

Dairy Products: In general, the following dairy products are right for your soul

- Kefir
- Full fat yogurt
- Full fat raw cheese
- Full fat cottage cheese
- Heavy whipping cream
- Full fat sour cream
- Full fat cream cheese
- Ghee
- Butter

Drinks: All types of sweet or aerated drinks are to be entirely avoided in your Keto diet. Drink of plenty of water though! Good drinks include:

- Coconut milk
- Almond milk
- Cashew milk
- Broth and soups
- Herbal teas
- Coffee teas
- Water
- Seltzer water

- Club soda
- Lemon and lime juices
- Sparkline water
- Water

Nuts and Seeds: In general nuts and seeds are allowed, but you should try to keep your intake at low levels since they enhance your carbohydrate intake. Be cautious while consuming nuts. However, keep In mind that you are to avoid peanuts as they fall under the legume category.

The following are allowed though:

- Almonds
- Macadamias
- Hazelnuts
- Pecans
- Pistachios
- Pine nuts
- Pumpkin seeds
- Sesame seeds
- Psyllium seeds
- Sunflower seeds
- Cashew nuts
- Walnuts
- Chia seeds

Herbs And Spices: As for herbs and spices, you are allowed to experiment with a wide variety of spices and herbs to enhance the flavor of your meals. Just make sure to avoid store-bought spices and herb that have hidden sugars of MSG's as they would break your Keto diet.

Recommended spices include:

- Black pepper
- White pepper
- Sea salt
- Basil
- Chili powder
- Curry powder
- Italian seasoning
- Cumin powder
- Oregano
- Thyme

- Sage
- Rosemary
- Turmeric
- Parsley
- Cilantro
- Cinnamon
- Cloves
- Allspices
- Paprika
- Ginger
- Cardamom

Awesome benefits of Ketogenic Diet

There are hundreds of different benefits that you can enjoy from a Ketogenic Diet! The following are just some of the benefits that you will experience in the long run:

Allows you to maintain weight effortlessly: Let's start off with the obvious one first. Yes, a Ketogenic diet will help you to lose weight by turning your body into a mean fat burning machine!

This would mean that the amount of effort needed for you to maintain your dream figure would be significantly reduced as your body will keep burning body throughout the whole day!

If you are an active person and like to exercise a lot, then the result of your physicals activities will be significantly improved as well!

Improve your Sleep Cycle: If you adopt the Ketogenic diet correctly, then you will enjoy a more sound sleep. Many Keto followers have reported that they were able to get a proper sleep without any interruption whatsoever. These improvements are strongly linked to the fact that you are limiting your daily glucose intake, which tends to facilitated lower levels of chronic inflammation in your body, which further allows your body to stay in a deep rest.

Stabilize Mood: As the number of Ketones increase in your body, it will help your body stabilize itself by controlling the various neurotransmitters such as dopamine and serotonin. Meaning, you will feel more cheerful and happy throughout the day with fewer amounts of sudden mood swings.

Will help you to deal with some different metabolic syndromes: Metabolic Syndrome refers to a type of medical condition that increases the risk of your suffering from heart diseases or diabetes.

Some syndromes include:

- Abdominal obesity
- High blood pressure
- Low HDL cholesterol levels
- High triglycerides
- High blood sugar levels

Will give you bursts of energy: Generally speaking, Ketones are excellent sources of energy, and they will help to keep your body energized all throughout the day! This will help you fend off chronic fatigue syndromes and save you from the "Sugar Rush" effect.

It will help you deal with some different diseases: Studies have shown that a Ketogenic diet helps to deal with a large number of different diseases. These include Alzheimer's, depression, Polycystic Ovary Syndrome, Stroke, Brain injury and so on.

One of the deadliest forms of disease of our current generation, "Cancer" is nowadays also seen as a disease that can be tackled through a Ketogenic diet.

Scientists believe that with proper and methodical treatment, a Ketogenic Diet can "Starve" the cancerous cells to death and destroy them in the process.

And those are just some of the benefits that you will enjoy in the long run!

Hearty tips for success

It is extremely crucial for you that you keep the following tips in mind to ensure that you able unlock the full potential of your diet.

- Make sure to go through your pantry and get rid of all high carb ingredients and foods before starting your Keto journey.

- Try to follow the Ketogenic diet with a friend or another family member. It will help you stay encouraged and inspired all throughout the journey

- Make sure to eat a sufficient amount of food and maintaining the levels of fat, protein, and carbs as needed

- Try to make dishes that you will enjoy! Being on a diet might be difficult if you are not enjoying it. There are a plethora of recipes that you can choose for your Ketogenic diet, so make your meal plan accordingly.

- Try to maintain a checklist or something similar to track your progress

- Make sure to keep your sodium intake in check to avoid future problems during your Ketogenic journey. Easy steps may include
  - ✓ Drinking organic broth if possible
  - ✓ Taking a just a pinch of pink salt with you consumed meals
  - ✓ Adding about ¼ teaspoon of pink salt to 16 ounces of water consumed
  - ✓ Adding vegetables such as kelp to your dishes
  - ✓ Eating up vegetables such as cucumber or celery for a more natural approach to sodium replenishment

- It is essential to maintain a proper exercise routine to make sure that your body is in tip-top shape all throughout the regime.

- Try to buy a counter to keep track of your carbs.

- Make sure to keep yourself packed with a right amount of water to replenish flushed electrolytes

Mistakes to avoid early on

If you are a novice in the field of Ketogenic Diet, it is incredibly reasonable that you might make some mistakes early on. The following are some of the most common mistakes that people seem to make early on.

Losing patience: This is extremely crucial and is a deal breaker for many! You should keep in mind that a Ketogenic Diet won't bear results overnight, and it will take some time. So, don't lose your patience and prepare yourself for the journey ahead.

Not drinking enough water: Without drinking a right amount of water, your body won't be able to do what it's supposed to do correctly! You have to drink more water than you used to during a Keto diet to ensure that your whole body is working correctly. A general rule of thumb is to drink at least 0.5 to 1 ounces of water per pound of your body weight per day.

Comparing yourself to others: This is one of the biggest mistakes that individuals tend to make! You should appreciate the fact that every single individual's body reacts differently to dietary changes and some people progress faster than others. You should not feel disheartened by seeing that your friend is losing weight faster than you! Remember, slow and steady wins the race.

Not getting proper sleep: Just like water, your body requires a right amount of sleep; otherwise it will fall into a state of fatigue, making you feel lethargic all throughout the day.

Not preparing a meal plan: Meal Planning or prepping is something that individuals often ignore, but it is essential! Those who do not make a proper meal plan, often end up failing to accurately follow the diet and end up being hungry and overeating! Therefore, a Meal Plan is crucial as it will save you from these frustrations.

Chapter 2: Simple 7 Days Meal Plan

Week 1	Breakfast	Lunch	Dinner
Day 1 (Sunday)	The Easy And Creative Lemon Artichokes	The Assorted Turkey And Veggie Delight	Broccoli And Beef Mix
Day 2 (Monday)	The Amazing "Zero Crust" Kale And Mushroom Quiche	Hearty Chicken Curry	Lime And Cilantro Mix
Day 3 (Tuesday)	The Winning Bacon And Kale	Coconut And Pork Dish	Rosemary Flavored Pork Roast
Day 4 (Wednesday)	The Easy And Creative Lemon Artichokes	The Assorted Turkey And Veggie Delight	Broccoli And Beef Mix
Day 5 (Thursday)	The Amazing "Zero Crust" Kale And Mushroom Quiche	Hearty Chicken Curry	Lime And Cilantro Mix
Day 6 (Friday)	The Winning Bacon And Kale	Coconut And Pork Dish	Rosemary Flavored Pork Roast
Day 7 (Saturday)	The Easy And Creative Lemon Artichokes	The Assorted Turkey And Veggie Delight	Lime And Cilantro Mix

Reference for Weekly Shopping

For Breakfast

Recipe 1: The Easy And Creative Lemon Artichokes

- 5 large artichokes
- 1 teaspoon sea salt
- 2 stalks celery, sliced
- 2 large carrots, cut into matchsticks
- Juice from ½ a lemon
- ¼ teaspoon black pepper
- 1 teaspoon dried thyme
- 1 tablespoons dried rosemary
- Lemon wedges for garnish

Recipe 2: The Amazing "Zero Crust" Kale And Mushroom Quiche

- 6 large eggs
- 2 tablespoons unsweetened almond milk
- 2 ounces low –fat feta cheese, crumbled
- ¼ cup parmesan cheese, grated
- 1 and ½ teaspoons Italian seasoning
- 4 ounces mushrooms, sliced
- 2 cups kale, chopped

Recipe 3: The Winning Bacon And Kale

- 2 tablespoons bacon fat
- 2 pounds kale, rinsed and chopped
- 2 bacon slices, cooked and chopped
- 2 teaspoons garlic, minced
- 2 cups vegetable broth
- Salt and pepper to taste

For Lunch

Recipe 1: The Assorted Turkey And Veggie Delight

- 8 ounces baby carrots
- 2 fennel bulbs, sliced
- 8 ounces pearl onions
- 8 ounces button mushrooms
- 1 teaspoon dried thyme
- 1 teaspoon dried rosemary
- 1 teaspoon salt
- ¼ teaspoon fresh ground black pepper
- Zest of 1 lemon
- 1 whole turkey breast, skin on

Recipe 2: Hearty Chicken Curry

- 10 bone-in chicken thighs, skinless
- 1 cup sour cream
- 2 tablespoons. Curry powder
- 1 onion, chopped
- 1 jar (16 ounces) chunky salsa sauce

Recipe 3: Coconut And Pork Dish

- 2 tablespoons coconut oil
- 4 pounds boneless pork shoulder, cut into 2 inch pieces
- Salt and pepper to taste
- 1 large onion, chopped
- 3 tablespoons garlic cloves, minced
- 3 tablespoons fresh ginger, minced
- 1 tablespoon curry powder
- 1 tablespoon ground cumin
- ½ teaspoon ground turmeric
- 1 cup unsweetened coconut milk
- Chopped cilantro, green onions for garnish

For Dinner

Recipe 1: Lime And Cilantro Chicken Mix

- 2 small limes
- ¼ cup cilantro, chopped
- ½ tablespoon fresh garlic, minced
- 1 teaspoon salt
- ½ teaspoon pepper
- 4 pounds chicken drumsticks

Recipe 2: Rosemary Flavored Pork Roast

- 3 pounds pork shoulder roast
- 1 cup bone broth
- 6 sprigs fresh rosemary
- 4 sprigs basil leaves
- 1 tablespoon chives, chopped
- ¼ teaspoon ground black pepper
- 3 organic pink lady apples, chopped

Recipe 3: Broccoli And Beef Mix

- 1 and ½ pounds beef round steak, cut into 2 inch by 1/8 inch strips
- 1 cup broccoli, diced
- ½ teaspoon red pepper flakes
- 2 teaspoon garlic, minced
- 2 teaspoons olive oil
- 2 tablespoons apple cider vinegar
- 2 tablespoons coconut aminos
- 2 tablespoons white wine vinegar
- 1 tablespoons arrowroot
- ¼ cup beef broth

Chapter 3: Breakfast Recipes

One Pan Breakfast

Serving: 4

Prep Time: 15 minutes

Ingredients

- 8 slices bacon
- 4 pcs. free-range eggs
- 1 medium-sized carrots julienned
- ½ cup celery, chopped
- ½ cup cauliflower, chopped
- 1 small white onion, chopped
- ½ cup gouda cheese, shredded
- 1 tbsp. butter

Directions

1. Prepare the vegetables and bacon.
2. Heat a large pan over medium fire and add the 1 tbsp. butter to melt.
3. Throw in the chopped vegetables and bacon and sauté for 20 mins or until the bacon is almost crisp. Remember to stir often.
4. Using a spatula, spread the vegetables and bacon evenly on the pan and then create four well.
5. Take one egg and then break it into the well. Do the same for the rest of the eggs.
6. Cover the pan with a lid and then heat until the eggs are cooked to your liking.
7. Turn off the heat and then sprinkle with the shredded cheese. Serve.

Nutritional Values

- Calories: 385 kcal
- Fat: 33.05g
- Carbohydrates: 5.58g

- Protein: 16.19g
- Dietary Fiber: 1.2g
- Cholesterol: 629mg

The Easy And Creative Lemon Artichokes

Serving: 4

Prep Time: 10 minutes

Cooking Time: 5 hours

Ingredients:

- 5 large artichokes
- 1 teaspoon sea salt
- 2 stalks celery, sliced
- 2 large carrots, cut into matchsticks
- Juice from ½ a lemon
- ¼ teaspoon black pepper
- 1 teaspoon dried thyme
- 1 tablespoons dried rosemary
- Lemon wedges for garnish

Directions:

1. Remove the stalk from your artichokes and remove tough outer shell

2. Transfer the chokes to your Slow Cooker and add 2 cups of boiling water

3. Add celery, lemon juice, salt, carrots, black pepper, thyme, rosemary

4. Cook on HIGH for 4-5 hours

5. Serve the artichokes with lemon wedges

6. Serve and enjoy!

Nutritional Contents:

- Calories: 205
- Fat: 2g
- Carbohydrates: 12g
- Protein: 34g

Lovely Teriyaki Chicken Platter

Serving: 6

Prep Time: 10 minutes

Cooking Time: 8 hours

Ingredients:

- 2 and ½ pounds skinless chicken breast
- 1 cup low sodium chicken broth
- 2 ounces pepperoncini with liquid
- 2 tablespoons Italian seasoning

Directions:

1. Add all of the listed ingredients to the slow cooker
2. Cook on LOW for 4 hours
3. Once done, slice up the chicken and serve!

Nutritional Contents:

- Calories: 379
- Fat: 2g
- Carbohydrates: 14g
- Protein: 71g

The Amazing "Zero Crust" Kale And Mushroom Quiche

Serving: 6

Prep Time: 10 minutes

Cooking Time: 8-9 hours

Ingredients:

- 6 large eggs
- 2 tablespoons unsweetened almond milk
- 2 ounces low –fat feta cheese, crumbled
- ¼ cup parmesan cheese, grated
- 1 and ½ teaspoons Italian seasoning
- 4 ounces mushrooms, sliced
- 2 cups kale, chopped

Directions:

1. Grease the inner pot of your Slow Cooker
2. Take a large bowl and whisk in eggs, cheese, almond milk, seasoning and mix it well
3. Stir in kale and mushrooms
4. Pour the mix into Slow Cooker
5. Gently stir
6. Place lid and cook on LOW for 8-9 hours
7. Serve and enjoy!

Nutritional Contents:

- Calories: 112
- Fat: 7g
- Carbohydrates: 4g
- Protein: 10g

The Winning Bacon And Kale

Serving: 4

Prep Time: 15 minutes

Cooking Time: 6 hours

Ingredients:

- 2 tablespoons bacon fat
- 2 pounds kale, rinsed and chopped
- 2 bacon slices, cooked and chopped
- 2 teaspoons garlic, minced
- 2 cups vegetable broth
- Salt and pepper to taste

Directions:

1. Grease inner pot with bacon fat
2. Add kale, garlic, bacon and broth to insert and toss to coat
3. Cover and cook on LOW for 6 hours
4. Season with salt and pepper
5. Serve and enjoy!

Nutritional Contents:

- Calories: 147
- Fat: 10g
- Carbohydrates: 7g
- Protein: 7g

HeartThrobe Broccoli Casserole

Serving: 4

Prep Time: 15 minutes

Cooking Time: 6 hours

Ingredients:

- 1 tablespoon extra-virgin olive oil
- 1 pound broccoli, cut into florets
- 1 pound cauliflower, cut into florets
- ¼ cup almond flour
- 2 cups coconut milk
- ½ teaspoon ground nutmeg
- Pinch of fresh ground black pepper
- 1 and ½ cups cashew cream

Directions:

1. Grease the Slow Cooker inner pot with olive oil
2. Place broccoli and cauliflower to your Slow Cooker
3. Take a small bowl and stir in almond flour, coconut milk, pepper, 1 cup of cashew cream
4. Pour coconut milk mixture over vegetables and top casserole with remaining cashew cream
5. Cover and cook on LOW for 6 hours
6. Server and enjoy!

Nutritional Contents:

- Calories: 377
- Fat: 32g
- Carbohydrates: 12g
- Protein: 16g

Simple Smoked Salmon And Spinach Frittata

Serving: 4

Prep Time: 15 minutes

Cooking Time: 8 hours

Ingredients:

- 10 whole eggs
- ¼ cup unsweetened almond milk
- 1 teaspoon garlic powder
- 1 teaspoon orange-chili-garlic sauce
- ½ teaspoon sea salt
- ¼ teaspoon freshly ground black pepper
- 8 ounces smoked salmon, flaked
- 8 ounces shiitake mushrooms, sliced
- 2 cups baby spinach
- Oil for greasing

Directions:

1. Take a large sized bowl and add eggs, orange chili garlic sauce, almond milk, garlic powder and season with salt and pepper
2. Fold in smoked salmon, spinach and mushrooms
3. Mix well
4. Grease Slow Cooker with oil
5. Pour egg mix in Slow Cooker
6. Close lid and cook on LOW for 8 hours
7. Serve and enjoy!

Nutritional Contents:

- Calories: 176
- Fat: 9g
- Carbohydrates: 7g
- Protein: 17g

Cheesy Sausage Pie

Serving: 4

Prep Time: 8 minutes

Ingredients

- ¾ cup plus 2 tbsp. cheddar cheese, grated
- 2 pcs. chicken sausages
- ¼ cup coconut flour
- ¼ tsp. baking soda
- ½ tsp rosemary
- ¼ tsp. cayenne
- A pinch of kosher salt
- 5 egg yolks (free range)
- ¼ cup coconut oil
- 2 tbsp. coconut milk
- 2 tsp. lime juice

Directions

1. Preheat oven at 350F.
2. Slice the chicken sausages into small chunks and place on a heated skillet greased with butter.
3. While waiting for the sausages to cook, combine the ¼ cup cheddar, coconut flour, baking soda, rosemary, cayenne, and salt in a mixing bowl.
4. In a separate bowl, mix the yolks, coconut oil, coconut milk, and lime juice. Stir well.
5. Gradually add the wet ingredients into the bowl with the dry ingredients and fold to incorporate all the ingredients together.
6. Pour the mixture into 2 ramekins and add the cooked sausages also in the ramekins.
7. Place in the oven to cook for 25 minutes or until the pies turn light brown.
8. Add the remaining cheddar on top of the pies and place back in the oven to melt the cheese for 4-5 minutes. Serve.

Nutritional Values

- Calories: 613 kcal
- Fat: 55.06g
- Carbohydrates: 5.39g
- Protein: 24.84g
- Dietary Fiber : 0.4g
- Cholesterol: 1562mg

Bread-Free Sandwich

Serving: 2

Prep Time: 8 minutes

Ingredients

- 4 large free-range eggs
- 2 slices of pre-cooked ham
- 4 tbsp. provolone cheese, cut into thick slices
- A dash of Sriracha sauce
- A pinch of salt and pepper to taste
- 1 tbsp. butter

Directions

1. Melt the butter on a non-stick pan over medium fire. Crack the eggs, season with salt and pepper and fry until over easy.
2. Sandwich the slices of ham and cheese in between 2 cooked eggs.
3. Add a dash of Sriracha for an added kick (optional) and serve.

Nutritional Values

- Calories: 253 kcal

- Fat: 17.96g

- Carbohydrates: 6.9g

- Protein: 15.99g

- Dietary Fiber : 0.3g

- Cholesterol: 399mg

Pesto And Eggs

Serving: 3

Prep Time: 15 minutes

Ingredients

- 1 ½ tbsp. pesto sauce
- 4 free-range eggs
- 2 tbsp. butter
- 3 tbsp. source cream

Directions

1. Whisk the eggs in a bowl. You can lightly season it with salt and pepper.
2. Heat a non-stick pan over medium fire. Melt the butter and then pour the whisked egg on the hot pan.
3. Add the pesto sauce to the pan and stir.
4. Turn off the heat and then add the 3 scoops of sour cream. Stir well.
5. You can serve with on the side of a mashed avocado.

Nutritional Values

- Calories: 210 kcal

- Fat: 22.46g

- Carbohydrates: 1.31g

- Protein: 1.9g

- Dietary Fiber : 0.1g

- Cholesterol: 47mg

Ketogenic Pancakes

Serving: 2

Prep Time: 10 minutes

Ingredients

- 4 large free-range eggs
- ¾ cup nut butter
- ½ tsp. baking soda
- 1 tsp. cinnamon powder
- 1/3 cup coconut milk
- 2 tbsp. of a sugar substitute like stevia or erythritol
- 2 tbsp. butter or clarified butter

Directions

1. Add all the ingredients in a food processor (except the 2 tbsp. butter) and pulse until all the ingredients are thoroughly combined. Set aside.
2. Melt the butter on a non-stick pan over low fire. Scoop ¼ cup of the pancake batter into the hot pan and then cook until the pancake has set, flip and cook until finished.
3. Repeat the same procedure for the rest of the batter. You can serve this with a drizzle of an all-natural maple syrup.

Nutritional Values

- Calories: 329 kcal
- Fat: 29.11g
- Carbohydrates: 13.32g
- Protein: 7.39g
- Dietary Fiber : 1.4g
- Cholesterol: 161mg

Heavenly Cakes

(Prep Time: 20 MIN| Serve: 3)

Serving: 3

Prep Time: 20 minutes

Ingredients

- 6 free-range eggs
- 350 grams ham, cooked and cut into cubes
- 1 yellow onion, chopped
- 2 tbsp. onion chopped chives
- 1 cup shredded cheddar
- 3 tbsp. plus 1 tbsp. butter
- ½ cup heavy cream

Directions

1. Preheat the oven at 400F.
2. Melt the 3 tbsp. butter in a skillet heated over medium fire.
3. Add the onions to the pan and sauté until the onions are translucent. Add the garlic and sauté for another minute or two. Turn off the heat and transfer the in a large bowl.
4. Add the rest of the ingredients in the bowl with the sautéed vegetables except for the 1 tbsp. butter. Stir well and set aside.
5. Take 6 pcs. of ramekins and brush it with the 1 tbsp. butter. Pour the mixture into the prepared ramekins filling only ½ of the cups.
6. Place in the oven to cook for 20 minutes or until the top turns light brown. Serve.

Nutritional Values

- Calories: 420 kcal

- Fat: 31.87g

- Carbohydrates: 7.55g

- Protein: 25.52g
- Dietary Fiber : 0.7g
- Cholesterol: 1291mg

All-In Omelet

Serving: 2

Prep Time: 5 minutes

Ingredients

- 4 eggs whites from a free range egg
- 1 pc. yolk
- 1 pc. heirloom tomato, chopped
- 1 cup baby spinach, roughly chopped
- ¼ cup cheddar, shredded
- 1 small white onion, chopped
- ½ tsp. dried basil
- 2 tbsp. coconut milk
- 1 tbsp. butter

Directions

1. Place all the egg whites and yolk in a mixing bowl. Add the 2 tbsp. coconut milk and whisk all the ingredients together.
2. Melt the butter on a non-stick pan over medium fire. Throw in the baby spinach, cheddar, chopped tomato, and onion. Sauté for 5 minutes or until the spinach is wilted. Set aside.
3. Transfer the sautéed vegetables on a plate and set aside.
4. Pour the egg mixture into the same pan and cook the eggs until done.
5. Place the cooked egg on a serving plate and then top one half of the egg with the cooked vegetables. Fold the egg and to create an omelet. Serve.

Nutritional Values

- Calories: 601 kcal
- Fat: 33.57g
- Carbohydrates: 8.95g

- Protein: 25.29g
- Dietary Fiber : 1.5g
- Cholesterol: 1363mg

The Denver Omelet!

Serving: 3

Prep Time: 10 minutes

Cooking Time: 4-6 hours

Ingredients:

- 6 large eggs
- 1 tablespoon unsweetened almond milk
- 1 garlic clove, minced
- ½ teaspoon salt
- ¼ teaspoon freshly ground black pepper
- 8 ounces ham, diced
- 2 red/green bell peppers, seeded and diced
- 1 small onion, diced
- ¼ cup tomatoes, diced
- 2 cups shredded low-fat Cheddar cheese

Directions:

1. Grease the Slow Cooker with cooking spray
2. Take a large bowl and whisk in eggs, almond, almond milk, garlic, salt, pepper and mix well
3. Fold in ham, bell pepper, onions, tomatoes and 1 cup shredded cheese
4. Pour the mix in Slow Cooker
5. Place lid and cook on LOW for 4-6 hours until the eggs are set
6. Serve and enjoy!

Nutritional Contents:

- Calories: 518
- Fat: 33g
- Carbohydrates: 14g
- Protein: 45g

Chapter 4: Snacks Recipes

Hot Buffalo Wings

Serving: 8

Prep Time: 10 minutes

Cooking Time: 6 hours

Ingredients:

- 1 bottle of (12 ounce) hot pepper sauce
- ½ cup melted ghee
- 1 tablespoons dried oregano
- 2 teaspoons garlic powder
- 1 teaspoon onion powder
- 5 pounds chicken wing sections

Directions:

1. Take a large bowl and mix in hot sauce, ghee, garlic powder, oregano, onion powder and mix well
2. Add chicken wings and toss to coat
3. Pour mix into Slow Cooker and cook on LOW for 6 hours
4. Serve and enjoy!

Nutritional Contents:

- Calories: 529
- Fat: 4g
- Carbohydrates: 1g
- Protein: 31g

A Jar Full Of Pecans

Serving: 4

Prep Time: 10 minutes

Cooking Time: 2 hours

Ingredients:

- 3 cups of raw pecans
- ¼ cup of date paste
- 2 teaspoon of vanilla beans extract
- 1 teaspoon of sea salt
- 1 tablespoon of coconut oil

Directions:

1. Add all of the listed ingredients to your pot
2. Cook on LOW for about 3 hours, making sure to stir it from time to time
3. One done, allow it to cool and serve!

Nutritional Contents:

- Calories: 337
- Fat: 31g
- Carbohydrates: 16g
- Protein: 4g

Dressed Brussels

Serving: 4

Prep Time: 10 minutes

Cooking Time: 4-5 hours

Ingredients:

- 2 pounds Brussels, halved
- 2 red onions, sliced
- 2 tablespoons apple cider vinegar
- 1 tablespoon extra-virgin olive oil
- 1 teaspoon ground cinnamon
- ½ cup pecans, chopped

Directions:

1. Add Brussels and onions to Slow Cooker
2. Take a small bowl and add cinnamon, vinegar, olive oil
3. Pour mixture over sprouts and toss
4. Place lid and cook on LOW for 4-5 hours
5. Enjoy!

Nutritional Contents:

- Calories: 176
- Fat: 10g
- Carbohydrates: 14g
- Protein: 4g

The Exquisite Spaghetti Squash

Serving: 6

Prep Time: 5 minutes

Cooking Time: 7-8 hours

Ingredients:

- 1 spaghetti squash
- 2 cups water

Directions:

1. Wash squash carefully with water and rinse it well
2. Puncture 5-6 holes in the squash using a fork
3. Place squash in Slow Cooker
4. Place lid and cook on LOW for 7-8 hours
5. Remove squash to cutting board and let it cool
6. Cut squash in half and discard seeds
7. Use two forks and scrape out squash strands and transfer to bowl
8. Serve and enjoy!

Nutritional Contents:

- Calories: 52
- Fat: 0g
- Carbohydrates: 12g
- Protein: 1g

The Hearty Garlic And Mushroom Crunch

Serving: 6

Prep Time: 10 minutes

Cooking Time: 8 hours

Ingredients:

- ¼ cup vegetable stock
- 2 tablespoons extra virgin olive oil
- 1 tablespoon Dijon mustard
- 1 teaspoon dried thyme
- 1 teaspoon sea salt
- ½ teaspoon dried rosemary
- ¼ teaspoon fresh ground black pepper
- 2 pounds cremini mushrooms, cleaned
- 6 garlic cloves, minced
- ¼ cup fresh parsley, chopped

Directions:

1. Take a small bowl and whisk in vegetable stock, mustard, olive oil, salt, thyme, pepper and rosemary.

2. Add mushrooms, garlic and stock mix to your Slow Cooker.

3. Close lid and cook on LOW for 8 hours .

4. Open lid and stir in parsley.

5. Serve and enjoy!

Nutritional Contents:

- Calories: 92
- Fat: 5g
- Carbohydrates: 8g
- Protein: 4g

Juicy Garlic Chicken Livers

Serving: 4

Prep Time: 10 minutes

Cooking Time: 8 hours

Ingredients:

- 1 pound chicken livers
- 8 garlic cloves, minced
- 8 ounces cremini mushrooms, quartered
- 4 slices uncooked bacon, chopped
- 1 onion, chopped
- 1 cup bone broth
- 1 teaspoon dried thyme
- 1 teaspoon dried rosemary
- 1 teaspoon salt
- 1 teaspoon freshly ground black pepper
- ¼ cup fresh parsley, chopped

Directions:

1. Add livers, bacon, garlic, mushrooms, onion, thyme, broth, rosemary to Slow Cooker
2. Season with salt and pepper
3. Place lid and cook on LOW for 8 hors
4. Remove lid and stir in parsley
5. Serve and enjoy!

Nutritional Contents:

- Calories: 210
- Fat: 9g
- Carbohydrates: 6g
- Protein: 24g

Worthy Bacon-Wrapped Drumsticks

Serving: 6

Prep Time: 10 minutes

Cooking Time: 8 hours

Ingredients:

- 12 chicken drumsticks
- 12 slices thin-cut bacon

Directions:

1. Wrap each chicken drumsticks in bacon
2. Place drumsticks in your Slow Cooker
3. Place lid and cook on LOW for 8 hours
4. Serve and enjoy!

Nutritional Contents:

- Calories: 202
- Fat: 8g
- Carbohydrates: 3g
- Protein: 30g

Avocado Chocolate Pudding

Serving: 4

Prep Time: 10 minutes

Ingredients

- 1 tbsp. coconut milk
- 1 avocado
- 2½ tbsp. raw cocoa powder
- 1 pinch sea salt
- ½ tbsp. vanilla extract
- 1 tsp ceylon cinnamon
- 1 tbsp coconut sugar
- 1 pinch stevia
- 1/16 tsp ground cayenne pepper

Directions

1. Cut and pit the avocado into a blender.
2. Blend until smooth.
3. Add in the coconut milk, cocoa powder and vanilla extract. Blend until smooth.
4. Add in coconut sugar, cayenne pepper, stevia and cinnamon.
5. Continue blending and make sure that all the chunks are blended by scraping down the sides of the food processor.
6. Serve with sprinkle of sea salt on the pudding.

Nutritional Values
- Calories: 180 kcal
- Fat: 15g (84.9%)
- Carbohydrates: 3.5g (7.6%)
- Protein: 3g (7.5%)

Crunchy Kale Chips

Serving: 4

Prep Time: 15 minutes

Ingredients

- 1 tsp soy sauce
- 1 tps fish sauce
- 2 tbsp sriracha
- 2 tbsp olive oil
- 1 bunch of kale
- 1tsp of sea salt

Directions

1. Remove the kale from the stems
2. Preheat oven to 350 F
3. Line with parchment paper
4. Break it into chip sized pieces and placed it in a bowl.
5. Add sriracha, olive oil, soy sauce and fish sauce.
6. Swirl the mixture and pour the dressing over the kale leaves.
7. Place the leaves out on the parchment paper
8. Baked until crisp. Approx. 8 – 12 minutes.
9. Sprinkling the sea salt over the kale leaves
10. Serve it.

Nutritional Values

- Calories: 49 kcal
- Fat: 0.9g
- Carbohydrates: 9g
- Protein: 4.3g
- Dietary Fiber : 1g
- Cholesterol: 0mg

Granola Bars

Serving: 4

Prep Time: 25 minutes

Ingredients

- 2 eggs
- 1 tbsp. nut butter
- 2 tsp dried cinnamon
- 2 tbsp. cocoa nibs
- 1 tsp vanilla
- 50g shredded coconut
- 100g almonds
- 50g pumpkin seeds
- 50g linseed
- 50g sunflower seeds
- 50g pumpkin seeds
- 50g macadamia nuts
- 3 tbsp. stevia
- 50g coconut oil

Directions

1. Mix all the ingredients into the blender
2. Blend until smooth but little chunks of nuts and seeds are still visible.
3. Form 10 bars and place it on a dish with lined parchment paper
4. Bake at 350F until golden or for 20 minutes.

Nutritional Values

- Calories: 245 kcal
- Fat: 21g
- Carbohydrates: 7g
- Protein: 7g
- Dietary Fiber : 4.5g
- Cholesterol: 0mg

Pepper Sea Salt Pork Rinds

Serving: 3

Prep Time: 35 minutes

Ingredients

- Pinch sea salt
- Pepper
- 2 to 4 lbs pork back fat and skin
- coconut oil

Directions

1. Preheat oven to 250F
2. Slice the pork skin and fat into long strips carefully. A sharp knife is required.
3. Separate a portion of the fat from the skin from one end of the strip.
4. Slice further to remove remaining fat.
5. Cut each strip into squares.
6. Place the strip (fat-side) down, on the wire rack with a baking sheet beneath.
7. Bake until the skin is crisp. Approx. 3 hours.
8. Pour the coconut oil into the pan.
9. Heat up the oil.
10. Add the pork rinds and cook until they puff up. Approx. 3 – 5 minutes.
11. Drain on a paper towel-lined plate.
12. Serve with sprinkle of pepper and sea salt.

Nutritional Values

- Calories: 152 kcal
- Fat: 20g (100%)
- Carbohydrates: 0g
- Protein: 0g
- Dietary Fiber : 1g
- Cholesterol: 0mg

Salted Crispy Macadamia Nuts

Serving: 4

Prep Time: 15 minutes

Ingredients

- 3lb raw macadamia nuts
- 3 tbsp. sea salt
- filtered water

Directions

1. Mix the nuts and sea salt in a bowl and cover by 3 inches of water
2. Leave the bowl in a warm area for 8 hours.
3. Drain the nuts, and put them back in the bowl.
4. Add another few teaspoons of sea salt to season.
5. Place the nuts in your oven on lowest setting until dried out.

Nutritional Values

- Calories: 945kcal
- Fat: 100g
- Carbohydrates: 17g
- Protein: 10g
- Dietary Fiber : 11g
- Cholesterol: 0mg

Hard Boiled Egg

Serving: 2

Prep Time: 10 minutes

Ingredients

- 4 eggs

Directions

1. Place the eggs into a pot.
2. Cover it with water with the eggs submerge.
3. Boil over medium-high heat
4. Place lid over the pot
5. Remove and let it cool for 10 minutes.
6. Serve it.

Nutritional Values

- Calories: 202 kcal
- Fat: 14g
- Carbohydrates: 2g
- Protein: 17g
- Dietary Fiber : 0g
- Cholesterol: 373mg

Cheesy Bacon Wrap Sticks

Serving: 3

Prep Time: 25 minutes

Ingredients

- 4 slices of bacon
- coconut oil
- 2 mozzarella cheese sticks
- 1 egg

Directions

1. Beat the egg in a bowl
2. Slice the cheese stick into quarters.
3. Preheat coconut oil in deep fryer to 350 F
4. Dip the ends of the bacon into the bowl.
5. Wrap the cheese sticks with bacon.
6. Drop the bacon wrapped cheese into the deep fryer
7. Cook until the bacon is brown and crispy. Approx. 2 – 3 minutes.
8. Transfer over to a plate with paper towel.
9. Serve it.

Nutritional Values
- Calories: 113 kcal
- Fat: 9g
- Carbohydrates: 1g
- Protein: 7g
- Dietary Fiber : 0g
- Cholesterol: 0 mg

Fried Avocado With Lemon

Serving: 2

Prep Time: 8 minutes

Ingredients

- 1 avocado
- 1 tbsp. lemon juice
- 1 tbsp. coconut oil
- pinch of sea salt

Directions

1. Remove the seed and slice the avocado into pieces
2. Preheat the pan with coconut oil
3. Fry the avocado slices till gentle brown.
4. Sprinkle the lemon juice and sea salt over the slices.
5. Serve it.

Nutritional Values

- Calories: 180 kcal
- Fat: 18g
- Carbohydrates: 9g
- Protein: 3g
- Dietary Fiber : 7g
- Cholesterol: 0mg

Keto Meatballs

Serving: 2

Prep Time: 25 minutes

Ingredients

- 500g ground beef
- 2 eggs
- 1 tsp dried tyme
- 1 tsp sea salt
- 2 cloves garlic, minced
- 1 tsp dried oregano
- coconut flour
- 1 cup diced mozzarella
- freshly grounded black pepper
- ½ cup coconut flour

Directions

1. Preheat the over to 450F
2. Dice the mozzarella in 20 -25 square pieces
3. Place it in freezer for 45 - 60 minutes
4. Combine all the ingredients into a large bowl.
5. Mix and Stir with your clean hands
6. Roll the meat into 20 – 25 pieces
7. Remove the cheese from freezer
8. Wrap the meat over the cheese.
9. Roll between hands and placed it on the baking tray with parchment paper.
10. Bake for 13 – 15 minutes.
11. Serve it.

Nutritional Values

- Calories: 117kcal
- Fat: 9.3g
- Carbohydrates: 1.4g
- Protein: 7g
- Dietary Fiber : 0.5g
- Cholesterol: mg

Chapter 5: Meat Recipes

Amazing Lemon And Artichoke Chicken

Serving: 6

Prep Time: 10 minutes

Cooking Time: 8 hours

Ingredients:

- 1 pound boneless and skinless chicken breast
- 1 pound boneless and skinless chicken thigh
- 14 ounces (can) artichoke hearts, packed in water and drained
- 1 onion, diced
- 2 carrots, diced
- 3 garlic cloves, minced
- 1 bay leaf
- ½ teaspoon pepper
- 3 cups turnips, peeled and cubed
- 6 cups chicken broth
- 14 cup fresh lemon juice
- ¼ cup parsley, chopped

Directions:

1. Add the above mentioned ingredients to your cooker except lemon juice and parsley
2. Cook on LOW for 8 hours
3. Remove the chicken and shred it up
4. Return it back to the slow cooker
5. Season with some pepper and salt!
6. Stir in parsley and lemon juice and serve!

Nutritional Contents:

- Calories: 400
- Fat: 10g
- Carbohydrates: 12g
- Protein: 3g

Supreme Hungarian Chicken Dish

Serving: 6

Prep Time: 10 minutes

Cooking Time: 7-8 hours

Ingredients:

- 1 tablespoon extra-virgin olive oil
- 2 pounds boneless chicken thigh
- ½ cup chicken broth
- Juice and zest of 1 lemon
- 2 teaspoon garlic, minced
- 2 teaspoon paprika
- ½ teaspoon salt
- 1 cup cashew cream
- 1 tablespoon parsley, chopped

Directions:

1. Lightly grease the inner pot of your Slow Cooker with olive oil
2. Add chicken thigh to Slow Cooker
3. Take a bowl and add broth, lemon juice, garlic, paprika, zest and salt
4. Mix and pour the mixture over chicken
5. Cook on LOW for 7-8 hours
6. Remove heat and stir n cashew cream
7. Serve with a topping of parsley
8. Enjoy!

Nutritional Contents:

- Calories: 404
- Fat: 32g
- Carbohydrates: 4g
- Protein: 23g

The Assorted Turkey And Veggie Delight

Serving: 8

Prep Time: 15 minutes

Cooking Time: 8 hours

Ingredients:

- 8 ounces baby carrots
- 2 fennel bulbs, sliced
- 8 ounces pearl onions
- 8 ounces button mushrooms
- 1 teaspoon dried thyme
- 1 teaspoon dried rosemary
- 1 teaspoon salt
- ¼ teaspoon fresh ground black pepper
- Zest of 1 lemon
- 1 whole turkey breast, skin on

Directions:

1. Arrange the baby carrots, fennels, onions, mushrooms at the bottom of your Slow Cooker.
2. Take a small bowl and add thyme, salt, rosemary, lemon zest and pepper.
3. Rub the outside of your Turkey with the mixture .
4. Place turkey in Slow Cooker and top with veggies.
5. Cover and cook on LOW for 8 hours.
6. Serve and enjoy!

Nutritional Contents:

- Calories: 347
- Fat: 3g
- Carbohydrates: 10g
- Protein: 60g

Evergreen Pork Chop

Serving: 4

Prep Time: 10 minutes

Cooking Time: 4 hours

Ingredients:

- 6-8 boneless pork chops
- ¼ cup arrowroot flour
- 2 teaspoons dry mustard
- 1 teaspoon garlic powder
- 1 and ½ cups beef stock
- Cooking fat
- Salt and pepper to taste

Directions:

1. Take a bowl and add flour, garlic powder, black pepper, dry mustard and salt

2. Coat the pork chop with the mixture and keep any extra flour on the side

3. Take a skillet and place it over medium-high heat

4. Add cooking fat and allow the fat to melt

5. Brown the chops for 1-2 minutes per side and transfer to your Slow Cooker

6. Add beef stock to the flour mix and mix well

7. Pour the beef stock mix to the chops and place lid

8. Cook on HIGH for 3 hours

9. Enjoy!

Nutritional Contents:

- Calories: 118
- Fat: 6g
- Carbohydrates: 1g
- Protein: 13g

Hearty Chicken Curry

Serving: 4

Prep Time: 10 minutes

Cooking Time: 10 hours

Ingredients:

- 10 bone-in chicken thighs, skinless
- 1 cup sour cream
- 2 tablespoons. Curry powder
- 1 onion, chopped
- 1 jar (16 ounces) chunky salsa sauce

Directions:

1. Add chicken thigh to your Slow Cooker
2. Add onions, salsa, curry powder over chicken , stir and place lid
3. Cook on LOW for 10 hours
4. Open lid and transfer chicken to serving platter
5. Pour sour cream into sauce (cooking liquid) in the Slow Cooker
6. Stir well and pour the sauce over chicken
7. Serve!

Nutritional Contents:

- Calories: 400
- Fat: 20g
- Carbohydrates: 17g
- Protein: 39g

Coconut And Pork Dish

Serving: 4

Prep Time: 10 minutes

Cooking Time: 4 hours

Ingredients:

- 2 tablespoons coconut oil
- 4 pounds boneless pork shoulder, cut into 2 inch pieces
- Salt and pepper to taste
- 1 large onion, chopped
- 3 tablespoons garlic cloves, minced
- 3 tablespoons fresh ginger, minced
- 1 tablespoon curry powder
- 1 tablespoon ground cumin
- ½ teaspoon ground turmeric
- 1 cup unsweetened coconut milk
- Chopped cilantro, green onions for garnish

Directions:

1. Take a large sized skillet and add coconut oil
2. Allow it to heat up and add pork in batches, brown them and season with a bit of salt and pepper
3. Transfer to a Slow Cooker
4. Making sure that there's 2 tablespoon of worth of fat in the skillet, add onion, garlic, ginger, cumin, curry, turmeric and cook over low heat for 5 minutes
5. Add the mix to your Slow Cooker and place the lid
6. Cook on LOW for 4 hours
7. Serve with a garnish of cilantro and scallions
8. Enjoy!

Nutritional Contents:

- Calories: 231
- Fat: 17g
- Carbohydrates: 5g

- Protein: 14g

Fascinating Beef Casserole

Serving: 6

Prep Time: 10 minutes

Cooking Time: 8 hours

Ingredients:

- ½ cabbage, roughly sliced
- 1 onion, diced
- 3 cloves garlic, chopped
- 1 and ½ pounds ground beef
- 2 cups cauliflower rice
- 4 tablespoons Ghee
- 1 heaping tablespoon Italian seasoning
- ½ teaspoon crushed red pepper
- Salt and pepper to taste
- ½ cup fresh parsley, chopped

Directions:

1. Add the listed ingredients to your Slow Cooker (except parsley) and give it a nice stir
2. Place lid and cook on LOW for 7-8 hours until the beef is coked
3. Stir in parsley and serve
4. Enjoy!

Nutritional Contents:

- Calories: 320
- Fat: 18g
- Carbohydrates: 1g
- Protein: 17g

Lime And Cilantro Chicken Mix

Serving: 6

Prep Time: 5 minutes

Cooking Time: 2 hours 45 minutes

Ingredients:

- 2 small limes
- ¼ cup cilantro, chopped
- ½ tablespoon fresh garlic, minced
- 1 teaspoon salt
- ½ teaspoon pepper
- 4 pounds chicken drumsticks

Directions:

1. Juice the lime and add them to your cooker
2. Add ¼ cup of chopped cilantro, 1 teaspoon of salt, ½ a tablespoon of freshly minced garlic
3. Add the chicken drumsticks to the cooker and coat them well
4. Cover and cook for about 2 and a ½ hour of HIGH
5. Pre-heat your oven to a temperature of 500 degree Fahrenheit
6. Line up a cookie sheet with foil
7. Transfer the cooker drumstick from the cooker to the foil using tongs
8. Bake for 10 minutes until they are nicely browned, making sure to turn them halfway through
9. Serve with the cooking juices
10. Enjoy!

Nutritional Contents:

- Calories: 130
- Fat: 1g
- Carbohydrates: 2g
- Protein: 22g

Hearty Turkey With Garlic Sauce

Serving: 8

Prep Time: 10 minutes

Cooking Time: 8 hours

Ingredients:

- 5 large onions, thinly sliced
- 4 garlic cloves, minced
- ¼ cup white wine vinegar
- ½ teaspoon salt
- ¼ teaspoon ground black pepper
- ¼ teaspoon cayenne pepper
- 4 large skinless turkey thighs

Directions:

1. Gently lay the garlic and onions into the bottom of your pot.
2. Pour in some wine with a sprinkle of salt, cayenne pepper and black pepper.
3. Add turkey thighs and cover it up.
4. Let it cook on low settings for about 8 hours.
5. Remove the turkey from the crock pot and clean up the flesh from the bones.
6. Keep the lid open and keep cooking until the liquid has completely evaporated, making sure to stir from time to time
7. Return the turkey to the pot.
8. Nestle the turkey into the mix.
9. Serve hot.
10. Enjoy!

Nutritional Contents:

- Calories: 845
- Fat: 41g
- Carbohydrates: 7g
- Protein: 45g

Rosemary Flavored Pork Roast

Serving: 4

Prep Time: 10 minutes

Cooking Time: 8 hours

Ingredients:

- 3 pounds pork shoulder roast
- 1 cup bone broth
- 6 sprigs fresh rosemary
- 4 sprigs basil leaves
- 1 tablespoon chives, chopped
- ¼ teaspoon ground black pepper

Directions:

1. Add all of the listed Ingredients to a slow cooker .
2. Cook on LOW for about 8-10 hours .
3. Slice the roast into smaller pieces if preferred and serve!

Nutritional Contents:

- Calories: 248
- Fat: 8g
- Carbohydrates: 0.7g
- Protein: 39g

The Authentic Pork Chili Colorado

Serving: 6

Prep Time: 10 minutes

Cooking Time: 8 hours

Ingredients:

- 3 pounds pork shoulder, cut into 1 inch cubes
- 1 teaspoon garlic powder
- 1 onion, chopped
- 1 teaspoon chipotle chili powder
- 1 tablespoon chili powder
- 1 teaspoon sea salt

Directions:

1. Add listed ingredients to Slow Cooker, give it a nice stir
2. Place lid and cook on LOW for 8 hours
3. Serve and enjoy!

Nutritional Contents:

- Calories: 506
- Fat: 37g
- Carbohydrates: 2g
- Protein: 40g

Broccoli And Beef Mix

Serving: 6

Prep Time: 10 minutes

Cooking Time: 6-8 hours

Ingredients:

- 1 and ½ pounds beef round steak, cut into 2 inch by 1/8 inch strips
- 1 cup broccoli, diced
- ½ teaspoon red pepper flakes
- 2 teaspoon garlic, minced
- 2 teaspoons olive oil
- 2 tablespoons apple cider vinegar
- 2 tablespoons coconut aminos
- 2 tablespoons white wine vinegar
- 1 tablespoons arrowroot
- ¼ cup beef broth

Directions:

1. Take a large sized bowl and make the sauce by mixing in red pepper flakes, olive oil, coconut aminos, garlic, white wine vinegar, apple cider vinegar, broth and arrowroot
2. Mix well
3. Add the mix to your Slow Cooker
4. Add beef and place a lid
5. Cook on LOW for 6-8 hours
6. Remove lid just 30 minutes before end time and add broccoli, place lid and let it finish
7. Serve and enjoy!

Nutritional Contents:

- Calories: 208
- Fat: 12g
- Carbohydrates: 11g
- Protein: 15g

Standard Pork Roast

Serving: 4

Prep Time: 8 minutes

Cooking Time: 8 hours

Ingredients:

- 1 large red onion, sliced
- 2 garlic cloves, minced
- 1 cup water
- 2 pounds boneless pork loin roast
- 1 cup water
- 2 tablespoons red wine vinegar
- 2 tablespoons Worcestershire sauce
- ½ teaspoon salt
- ½ teaspoon pepper

Directions:

1. Arrange onion slices and minced garlic on the bottom of your Slow Cooker
2. Place the roast on top
3. Take a mixing bowl and add the rest of the ingredients, transfer the mixture over the roast
4. Cover with lid and cook on LOW for 8 hours
5. Serve and enjoy!

Nutritional Contents:

- Calories: 361
- Fat: 31g
- Carbohydrates: 8g
- Protein: 31g

Crowd Favorite Chicken Thighs

Serving: 4

Prep Time: 10 minutes

Cooking Time: 6-8 hours

Ingredients:

- 3 pounds boneless chicken thighs, skinless
- 2 tablespoons apple cider vinegar
- ½ cup agave nectar
- 2 teaspoon garlic powder
- 2 teaspoon paprika
- 1 teaspoon chili powder
- 1 teaspoon red pepper flakes
- 1 teaspoon black pepper
- 2 teaspoon salt

Directions:

1. Take a bowl and add garlic pepper, paprika, chili powder, red pepper flakes, salt and pepper

2. Take another bowl and mix in agave nectar, vinegar and keep the mix on the side

3. Use the seasoning mix to properly coat the chicken thigh

4. Pour nectar, vinegar mix over chicken

5. Transfer the mix to Slow Cooker

6. Place lid and cook on LOW for 6-8 hours

7. Drizzle the glaze on top and serve

8. Enjoy!

Nutritional Contents:

- Calories: 234
- Fat: 15g
- Carbohydrates: 14g
- Protein: 8g

Garlic And Tomato Chicken Herbs

Serving: 4

Prep Time: 10 minutes

Cooking Time: 5-7 hours

Ingredients:

- 3 pounds boneless, skinless chicken thighs
- ½ cup low-sodium chicken broth
- 2 cups cherry tomatoes, halved
- 4 garlic cloves, minced
- 2 teaspoons garlic salt
- ¼ teaspoon ground white pepper
- 2 tablespoons fresh basil, chopped
- 2 tablespoons fresh oregano, chopped

Directions:

1. Add listed ingredients to Slow Cooker
2. Gently stir
3. Cover with the lid and cook on LOW for 5-7 hours
4. Serve and enjoy!

Nutritional Contents:

- Calories: 247
- Fat: 5g
- Carbohydrates: 15g
- Protein: 34g

Beefy Tacos

Serving: 2

Prep Time: 25 minutes

Ingredients

- 1 lb. ground beef
- 2 tbsp. butter
- 3 cloves of garlic, minced
- 1 small onion, chopped
- 1 small can of green chilies
- 1 tsp. coriander, ground
- 2 tsp. chili powder
- ½ cups sour cream
- 2 cups cheddar cheese, grated
- Lettuce cups for the wrap

Directions

1. Melt the butter in a pan over medium fire and then sauté the onion and garlic until soft.
2. Add the ground beef and then cook until done.
3. Add the green chilies, coriander and chili powder. Mix well and allow to cook for 5 minutes.
4. Turn the heat to low and then add the sour cream and cheddar. Cook for another 15 minutes.
5. Scoop the prepared taco filling into lettuce cups and serve.

Nutritional Values

- Calories: 475 kcal
- Fat: 29.97g
- Carbohydrates: 14.22g
- Protein: 36.47g
- Dietary Fiber : 0.8g

- Cholesterol: 135mg

Beef Stir-Fry

Serving: 2

Prep Time: 20 minutes

Ingredients

- 1 ¼ lb. ground beef
- 1 tbsp. clarified butter
- 3 cloves of garlic
- ¼ tsp. ginger, minced
- 1 tsp. red pepper flakes
- ¼ cup coconut aminos
- ½ tsp. liquid stevia
- ½ tsp. molasses
- 2 pcs. green onions, chopped

Directions

1. Place a wok or skillet over medium fire. Melt the butter and then add the ground beef. Cook for a few minutes until brown.
2. Add the liquid stevia, coconut aminos, molasses and red pepper flakes and then stir and allow to simmer for 3-4 minutes.
3. Garnish with chopped green onions on top before serving.

Nutritional Values

- Calories: 324 kcal

- Fat: 20.93g

- Carbohydrates: 3.28g

- Protein: 29.15g

- Dietary Fiber : 0.7g

- Cholesterol: 106mg

Beef Balls In Creamy Sauce

Serving: 3

Prep Time: 15 minutes

Ingredients

- 1 ½ lb. ground beef
- 2 tbsp. Worcestershire sauce
- 3 tbsp. fresh parsley, chopped
- 3 cloves of garlic, minced
- 1 tsp. garlic powder
- 1 small onion, diced
- 1 tsp. onion powder
- Salt and pepper to taste
- 2 tbsp. clarified butter
- 2 tbsp. butter
- ½ cup sliced button mushrooms
- 1 cup low-sodium beef stock
- 2 tbsp. cooking sherry
- 2 tbsp. beef bouillon granules
- ¼ cup heavy cream
- ¾ cup sour cream

Directions

1. In a large bowl, mix together the ground beef, one clove of the minced garlic, chopped parsley, Worcestershire, garlic powder and onion powder. Season with salt and pepper. Combine the ingredients with your hands and then create 4 patties.
2. Heat the clarified butter in a pan over medium-high fire. Place the patties and sear for about 2 minutes on each side. Remove the patties and set aside.
3. Using the same pan, melt the butter and drizzle the cooking sherry. Lower the fire and add the diced onion, button mushrooms, and the rest of the minced garlic. Cook until the onions are caramelized.
4. Pour the beef stock into the pan and also add the bouillon granules.

5.   Add the heavy cream and sour cream into the pan, followed by the browned patties. Allow to simmer on low fire for 10 minutes. Serve.

Nutritional Values

- Calories: 714 kcal

- Fat: 48.49g

- Carbohydrates: 19.73g

- Protein: 49.25g

- Dietary Fiber : 1.1g

- Cholesterol: 210mg

Beefy, Gooey Cheese, Goodness

Serving: 2

Prep Time: 35 minutes

Ingredients

- 1 lb. ground beef
- 1 cup cheddar cheese, grated
- 1 cup baby spinach, chopped
- 1 small bell pepper, chopped
- 5 free-range eggs
- A dash of salt and pepper to taste

Directions

1. Set the oven at 350F.
2. Place the ground beef on a skillet and cook until brown.
3. Transfer the cooked beef on a mixing bowl and then add the baby spinach and red pepper. Combine well.
4. Place the beef and spinach mixture into a baking dish greased with butter making sure it is well distributed onto the dish.
5. On another bowl, whisk the eggs and season with salt and pepper.
6. Add the cheddar cheese on top of the beef and then followed by the whisked egg.
7. Place the in the oven to bake for 18-20 minutes. Allow to cool for a few minutes before cutting into squares and serving.

Nutritional Values

- Calories: 391 kcal

- Fat: 22.41g

- Carbohydrates: 7.61g

- Protein: 40.85g

- Dietary Fiber : 1.4g

- Cholesterol: 333mg

Beef Sausage And Bacon Pot

Serving: 2

Prep Time: 15 minutes

Ingredients

- 1 lb. beef sausage
- 8 pcs. bacon strips, chopped
- 2 cups broccoli florets
- ½ cup heavy cream
- 1 tbsp. Dijon mustard
- ¼ cup cheddar cheese, grated

Directions

1. Set oven at 350F.
2. Cut the sausages into chunks and place on a baking dish with the chopped bacon.
3. Also add the florets into the dish making sure they're equally distributed.
4. In a small bowl, combine the cream and mustard and pour on top of the meat and broccoli.
5. Finally, sprinkle the top of the dish with the grated cheese and bake in the oven for 35 minutes.
6. Serve.

Nutritional Values

- Calories: 768 kcal

- Fat: 58.96g

- Carbohydrates: 5.58g

- Protein: 46.81g

- Dietary Fiber : 8.3g

- Cholesterol: 42mg

Filet Mignon Steak

Serving: 2

Prep Time: 20 minutes

Ingredients

- 2 large (about 1.5 inch thick) filet mignon steaks, cut in half
- 2 tbsp. ghee
- A pinch of salt and pepper to taste

Directions

1. Set oven at 275F
2. Take a paper towel and pat dry the steaks and then season with salt and pepper.
3. Lay the steaks on a baking rack on top of a baking sheet lined with foil.
4. Place in the oven to broil for 30 minutes or until the meat registers at 90F.
5. Remove the steaks from the oven and then place on a skillet with ghee over high heat.
6. Cook the steaks for about 2 minutes on each side.
7. Reduce the heat to medium and then brown all sides for another 1 minute each.
8. Serve with your favorite steak sauce.

Nutritional Values

- Calories: 22 kcal

- Fat: 15.85g

- Carbohydrates: 1.06g

- Protein: 17.77g

- Dietary Fiber : 0.2g

- Cholesterol: 75mg

Curried Ground Beef

Serving: 2

Prep Time: 25 minutes

Ingredients

- 1 lb. ground beef
- 3 pcs. carrots, chopped
- 1 pc. large tomato, chopped
- 1 tsp. mustard seeds
- 1 onion, chopped
- A handful of curry leaves
- 4 cloves of garlic, minced
- ½ tsp. ginger, minced
- 1 tsp. coriander powder
- ¼ tsp. chili powder
- ½ tsp. turmeric
- ½ tsp. sea salt
- 2 tsp. masala
- 2 tbsp. ghee
- 1 can coconut milk
- ¼ cup water

Directions

1. Heat the ghee on a pan over medium fire.
2. Throw in the mustard seeds and wait until the seeds start to pop before adding the chopped onion and curry leaves.
3. Sauté for 3 minutes and then add the minced garlic and ginger. Stir and then add the rest of the spices.
4. Add the ground beef and cook until brown.
5. Add the chopped potato and carrots and pour the ¼ cup water. Cover and simmer for 5 minutes.
6. Pour in the coconut milk, stir and cook for 15 minutes, or until the veggies are soft.
7. Serve.

Nutritional Values

- Calories: 332 kcal

- Fat: 19.1g

- Carbohydrates: 13.9g

- Protein: 30.g

- Dietary Fiber : 3.1g

- Cholesterol: 100mg

Chapter 6: Fish And Seafood Recipes

Hearty Crab Soup

Serving: 4

Prep Time: 20 minutes

Cooking Time: 6-7 hours

Ingredients:

- 1 cup crab meat, cubed
- 1 tablespoon garlic, minced
- Salt as needed
- Red chili flakes as needed
- 3 cups vegetable broth
- 1 teaspoon salt

Directions:

1. Coat the crab cubes in lime juice and let them sit for a while
2. Add the all ingredients (including marinated crab meat) to your Slow Cooker and put lid
3. Cook on MEDIUM for 3 hours
4. Let it sit for a while
5. Remove lid and simmer the soup for 5 minutes more on LOW
6. Stir and check seasoning
7. Enjoy!

Nutritional Contents:

- Calories: 201
- Fat: 11g
- Carbohydrates: 12g
- Protein: 13g

Cooked Salmon Fillet

Serving: 4

Prep Time: 5 minutes

Cooking Time: 1 hour

Ingredients:

- 2 tablespoons Ghee
- 1 small onion, thinly sliced
- 1 cup water
- ½ cup vegetable
- 4 salmon fillets
- 1 tablespoon fresh lemon juice
- 1 sprig fresh dill
- Salt and pepper to taste
- 1 lemon, quartered, for garnish

Directions:

1. Grease the slow cooker with ghee
2. Add onion slices to your pot and pour water
3. Add chicken broth and set the pot to HIGH, cook for 30 minutes
4. Place fillets on top of the cooked onion and add lemon juice alongside fresh dill
5. Cover lid and cook on HIGH for 30 minutes more
6. Season with pepper and salt
7. Garnish with lemon and enjoy!

Nutritional Contents:

- Calories: 220
- Fat: 12g
- Carbohydrates: 14g
- Protein: 31g

The Low Carb Clam Chowder

Serving: 8

Prep Time: 15 minutes

Cooking Time: 4 hours 20 minutes

Ingredients:

- 13 slices bacon, thick cut
- 2 cups chicken broth
- 1 cup celery, chopped
- 1 cup onion, chopped
- 6 cups baby clams, with juice
- 2 cups heavy whipping cream
- 1 teaspoon salt
- 1 teaspoon ground thyme
- 1 teaspoon pepper

Directions:

1. Take a skillet and place it over medium heat, cook bacon until crispy

2. Drain and crumble the bacon

3. Chop onion, celery and add them to the pan

4. Once tender add veggies alongside remaining ingredients to your Slow Cooker

5. Place lid and cook on LOW for 4-6 hors

6. Serve and enjoy@

Nutritional Contents:

- Calories: 427
- Fat: 33g
- Carbohydrates: 5g
- Protein: 27g

Asparagus And Tilapia Dish

Serving: 4

Prep Time: 20 minutes

Cooking Time: 2 hours

Ingredients:

- 1 bunch asparagus
- 4-6 tilapia fillets
- 8-12 tablespoons lemon juice
- Pepper for seasoning
- Lemon juice for seasoning
- ½ tablespoons for clarified butter, for each fillet

Directions:

1. Cut single pieces of foil for the fillets
2. Divide the bundle of asparagus into even number depending on the number of your fillets
3. Lay the fillets on each of the piece of foil and sprinkle pepper and add a teaspoon of lemon juice
4. Add clarified butter and top with asparagus
5. Fold the foil over the fish and seal the ends
6. Repeat with all the fillets and transfer to cooker
7. Cook on HIGH for 2 hours
8. Enjoy!

Nutritional Contents:

- Calories: 229
- Fat: 10g
- Carbohydrates: 1g
- Protein: 28g

Amazing Poached Salmon

Serving: 4

Prep Time: 10 minutes

Cooking Time: 1 and ½ hours

Ingredients:

- 2 cups water
- 1 cup dry white wine
- 1 bay leaf
- 1 shallot, thinly sliced
- 1 lemon, thinly sliced
- 1 teaspoon kosher salt
- 1 teaspoon black peppercorns
- 5-6 sprigs fresh herbs
- 2 pounds salmon, skin on (4-6 fillets)
- Salt, black pepper, olive oil or lemon wedges for garnish

Directions:

1. Add wine, water, bay leaf, shallots, salt, peppercorns, herbs to Slow Cooker
2. Place lid and cook on HIGH for 30 minutes
3. Sprinkle salmon with salt and pepper
4. Arrange in cooker, skin side facing down
5. Cover with lid and cook on LOW for 45 minutes
6. Let it sit for a few hours and drizzle oil, season with garnish and enjoy!

Nutritional Contents:

- Calories: 504
- Fat: 30g
- Carbohydrates: 3g
- Protein: 46g

Mesmerizing Shrimp Scampi

Serving: 3

Prep Time: 20 minutes

Cooking Time: 2 hours 30 minutes

Ingredients:

- 1 cup chicken broth
- ½ cup white wine vinegar
- 2 tablespoons olive oil
- 2 teaspoon garlic, chopped
- 2 teaspoons garlic, minced
- 1 pound large raw shrimp

Directions:

1. Add chicken broth, lemon juice, white wine vinegar, olive oil, lemon juice, chopped garlic and fresh minced parsley
2. Add thawed shrimp (the ratio should be 1 pound of shrimp for ¼ cup of chicken broth)
3. Place lid and cook on LOW for 2 and a ½ hours
4. Serve and enjoy!

Nutritional Contents:

- Calories: 293
- Fat: 24g
- Carbohydrates: 4g
- Protein: 16g

Easy Salmon Salad With Avocado

Serving: 2

Prep Time: 15 minutes

Ingredients

- 1 pc. salmon fillet
- 1 pc. green onion, chopped
- 2 tbsp. lime juice
- ¼ cup keto mayo
- 2 tbsp. fresh dill
- 1 tbsp. ghee
- 1 avocado
- Pinch of salt and pepper

Directions

1. Set oven at 400F.
2. Lay the salmon fillet on a baking sheet lined with parchment paper. Drizzle with juice of lime and ghee on top.
3. Season the salmon with salt and pepper and place in the oven to bake for 25 minutes.
4. When cooked, pull the salmon meat using a fork and place in a bowl.
5. Add the mayo and green onions in the bowl and stir.
6. Mash the avocado and add to the salmon salad. Lightly toss the ingredients together and serve.

Nutritional Values

- Calories: 490 kcal
- Fat: 31.99g
- Carbohydrates: 30.21g
- Protein: 26.7g
- Dietary Fiber : 9.3g
- Cholesterol: 94mg

Salmon Fillets

Serving: 3

Prep Time: 25 minutes

Ingredients

- 1 lb. salmon fillet
- ¼ cup button mushrooms, chopped
- 1 clove of garlic, minced
- ½ cup scallions, chopped
- ¼ cup tamari
- ¼ tsp. rosemary
- ¼ tsp. thyme
- ¼ tsp. tarragon
- ¼ tsp. basil
- ¼ tsp. oregano
- ¼ tsp. ginger, ground
- 2 tbsp. butter

Directions

1. Set oven at 350F.
2. Place the fish fillet in a re-sealable plastic bag and pour over the tamari, coconut oil, as well as the herbs and spices. Shake the bag well to coat the fish with the sauce and marinate in the fridge for 4 hours.
3. When done marinating, place the salmon fillet on a baking sheet lined with foil and bake for at least 10 minutes.
4. Melt the butter on a pan over medium heat. Add the mushrooms and scallions into the pan and cook until tender.
5. Take the salmon out from the oven and pour over the sautéed mushrooms. Place the fish back in the oven to bake for another 10 mins. Serve.

Nutritional Values

- Calories: 323 kcal
- Fat: 18.62g
- Carbohydrates: 3.35g
- Protein: 34.46g

- Dietary Fiber : 0.8g
- Cholesterol: 122mg

Parmesan Crusted Fish

Serving: 2

Prep Time: 25 minutes

Ingredients

- 1 lb. cream dory fillet
- 2 tbsp. milk
- 1 egg
- ¼ cup parmesan cheese, grated
- 2 tbsp. almond flour
- ½ tsp. smoked paprika
- Pinch of salt and pepper to taste

Directions

1. Set the oven at 350F
2. Whisk the egg and milk together in a bowl.
3. In a re-sealable plastic bag combine all the dry ingredients and shake well.
4. Dip the fish fillet into the egg and milk mixture and place inside the plastic bag. Shake to cover the fillets with the breading.
5. Place the fish fillets on a baking sheet lined with foil and cook in the oven for 25 minutes.
6. Serve with lemon wedges on the side.

Nutritional Values

- Calories: 293 kcal
- Fat: 26.65g
- Carbohydrates: 6.99g
- Protein: 7.71g
- Dietary Fiber : 0.3g
- Cholesterol: 236mg

Fish In Orange Pecan Butter Sauce

Serving: 2

Prep Time: 35minutes

Ingredients

- 1 pc. trout fillet, skin on
- ½ cup pecan nuts, chopped
- 1 pc. orange, juiced and zested
- 2 tbsp. butter, divided
- 1 tbsp. parsley, chopped
- A pinch of salt and pepper to taste

Directions

1. Melt 1 tbsp. of butter on a cast iron skillet over medium fire.
2. Flavor the trout with salt and pepper and place on the hot pan with the skin side up.
3. Sear the fish for 3 minutes on the other side. Set aside.
4. Using the same pan, melt the remaining butter and add the chopped pecans for about a minute. Pour the orange juice and allow to simmer for 2 minutes.
5. Orange pecan sauce over the fish and sprinkle with the orange zest and chopped parsley. Serve.

Nutritional Values

- Calories: 350 kcal
- Fat: 33.01g
- Carbohydrates: 5.66g 65%)
- Protein: 10.87g
- Dietary Fiber : 2.8g
- Cholesterol: 38mg

Grilled Fish

Serving: 2

Prep Time: 35 minutes

Ingredients

- 1 lb. tilapia fillets
- 2 limes, juiced
- 1 tbsp. fresh parsley, chopped
- 1 tsp. dill
- ¼ tsp. smoked paprika
- A pinch of salt and pepper to taste
- 2 tbsp. butter

Directions

1. Place a fillet on top of one heavy duty foil.
2. Melt the butter in a saucepan heated over low fire. Pour the lemon juice, add the dill, parsley, salt and pepper.
3. Equally pour the butter on top of the fillets and season with paprika on top.
4. Wrap the fillets with the foil making sure it's secured. Cook on the grill for 5 minutes on each side.
5. Serve.

Nutritional Values

- Calories: 171 kcal
- Fat: 7.7g
- Carbohydrates: 3.06g
- Protein: 23.2g
- Dietary Fiber : 0.3g
- Cholesterol: 72mg

Buttered Shrimp

Serving: 2

Prep Time: 35 minutes

Ingredients

- 1 ½ lb. shrimp, peel and veins removed
- 2 tbsp. plus 6 tbsp. butter
- 4 cloves of garlic, minced
- 1 juice of lemon
- ¼ cup low-sodium chicken stock
- A pinch of salt and pepper
- 2 tbsp. fresh parsley, chopped

Directions

1. Place a skillet over medium fire and melt the butter.
2. Add the shrimps and season with salt and pepper. Stir and cook for about 3 minutes or until the shrimps turn pink. Set aside.
3. Using the same pan, sauté the garlic for 1 minute. Pour the chicken stock and juice of lemon and allow to simmer for 3-5 minutes.
4. Add the 6 tbsp. butter on to the pan and stir until it fully melts.
5. Add the shrimp back to the pan and toss to coat with the garlic butter sauce.
6. Garnish with chopped parsley on top before serving.

Nutritional Values
- Calories: 236 kcal
- Fat: 25.52
- Carbohydrates: 3.2g
- Protein: 35.79g
- Dietary Fiber : 0.3g
- Cholesterol: 490mg

Creamy Shrimp And Bacon Bowl

Serving: 2

Prep Time: 35 minutes

Ingredients

- ¼ lb. shrimps, peel and vein removed
- ¼ lb. smoked salmon, roughly chopped
- 4 bacon strips, roughly chopped
- 1 cup button mushrooms, sliced
- ½ cup coconut cream
- A pinch of salt and pepper

Directions

1. Cook the chopped bacon on a cast iron skillet over medium fire.
2. Add the sliced mushrooms when the bacon is almost crispy and then cook for another 5 minutes. Remember to stir constantly.
3. Add the salmon to the pan and cook for 2 minutes.
4. Then, add the deveined shrimp and allow to cook for another 2 minutes.
5. Pour the coconut cream on the pan and then set the heat to low fire. Allow to simmer for a minute.
6. Serve.

Nutritional Values
- Calories: 340 kcal
- Fat: 29g (86.5%)
- Carbohydrates: 3.5g
- Protein: 17g (4.5%)
- Dietary Fiber : 1g

Baked Sardines

Serving: 2

Prep Time: 35 minutes

Ingredients

- 800g sardines
- 1 tsp. kosher salt
- A pinch of black pepper
- 8 tbsp. extra virgin olive oil
- 4 tbsp. mint leaves, chopped
- 4 tsp. dried basil

Directions

1. Set the oven at 350F.
2. Season sardines with salt and pepper and place on a baking rack.
3. Bake in the oven for 10 minutes.
4. When done cooking, sprinkle the sardines with the mint leaves and basil and finally, drizzle with extra virgin olive oil.

Nutritional Values

- Calories: 482 kcal
- Fat: 40g (69.1%)
- Carbohydrates: 0.20g (0.2%)
- Protein: 40.01g (30.8%)
- Dietary Fiber : 0.22g

Tuna Salad

Serving: 2

Prep Time: 35 minutes

Ingredients

- 1 head of romaine lettuce
- 1 can tuna
- 2 hardboiled eggs, sliced
- 2 tbsp. chives, chopped
- 2 tbsp. mayonnaise
- 1 tbsp. lime juice
- 1 tbsp. olive oil
- Pinch of salt to taste

Directions

1. Tear the lettuce and place on a serving plate.
2. In a bowl, combine the tuna, mayo, lime juice, and olive oil. Season with salt and toss to coat the fish well with the dressing.
3. Serve the tuna on top of the bed of lettuce and top with the slices of egg on top.

Nutritional Values

- Calories: 996 kcal
- Fat: 45.83g
- Carbohydrates: 25.08g
- Protein: 59.75g
- Dietary Fiber : 13.7g
- Cholesterol: 1297mg

Salmon And Avocado Omelet

Serving: 2

Prep Time: 35 minutes

Ingredients

- 3 whole eggs
- 50g smoked salmon
- ½ avocado, sliced
- 2 tbsp. cream cheese
- 2 tbsp. chives, chopped
- 1 tbsp. butter
- A pinch of salt and pepper to taste

Directions

1. Whisk the eggs in a bowl and season with salt and pepper.
2. In a separate bowl, combine the cream cheese and chives together. Set aside.
3. Melt the butter in a non-stick pan over medium heat. Pour the egg and move the pan side to side. Cook until done.
4. Transfer the cooked egg into a plate and spread the cream cheese and chive mixture on top.
5. Add the smoked salmon on top along with the avocado slices. Fold to create an omelet.
6. Serve.

Nutritional Values
- Calories: 765 kcal
- Fat: 66.9g
- Carbohydrates: 13.3g
- Protein: 36.9g
- Dietary Fiber : 7.4g

Slow Cooked Lobster Bisque

Serving: 3

Prep Time: 35 minutes

Ingredients

- 4 pcs. lobster tails
- 1 clove of garlic
- 2 pcs. shallots, minced
- ¼ cup fresh parsley leaves, chopped
- 1 tsp. dill
- ½ tsp. smoked paprika
- ¼ tsp. ground pepper
- 2 cups heavy cream
- 4 cups low-sodium chicken broth
- 1 can diced tomatoes (with juice)

Directions

1. Place the minced garlic and shallot in a bowl and microwave on high for 2 minutes.
2. Transfer into a slow cooker and then add the rest of the ingredients except for the lobster tails and heavy cream.
3. Cut the end of the lobster tail and then add to the crockpot. Cook on high for 3 hours.
4. When done cooking, remove the lobster tails from the pot and use an immersion blender to puree the soup. This depends on the consistency you prefer your bisque to be.
5. Add the lobster back into the pot and cook for another 45 minutes.
6. Remove again the lobster and chop.
7. Pour the heavy cream into the pot along with the chopped lobster. Stir well and serve hot.

Nutritional Values
- Calories: 505 kcal

- Fat: 24.96g
- Carbohydrates: 7.12g
- Protein: 31.44g
- Dietary Fiber: 1.2g
- Cholesterol: 273mg

Chapter 7: Vegetable Recipes

Easy Pepper Jack Cauliflower

Serving: 6

Prep Time: 10 minutes

Cooking Time: 3 hours 35 minutes

Ingredients:

- 1 head cauliflower
- ¼ cup whipping cream
- 4 ounces cream cheese
- ½ teaspoon pepper
- 1 teaspoon salt
- 2 tablespoons butter
- 4 ounces pepper jack cheese
- 6 bacon slices, crumbled

Directions:

1. Grease slow cooker and add listed ingredients (except cheese and bacon)
2. Stir and place lid, cook on LOW for 3 hours
3. Remove lid and add cheese, stir
4. Place lid and cook for 1 hour more
5. Garnish with bacon crumbles and enjoy!

Nutritional Contents:

- Calories: 272
- Fat: 21g
- Carbohydrates: 5g
- Protein: 10g

The Brussels Platter

Serving: 4

Prep Time: 15 minutes

Cooking Time: 4 hours

Ingredients:

- 1 pound Brussels sprouts, bottoms trimmed and cut
- 1 tablespoon olive oil
- 1 – ½ tablespoon Dijon mustard
- Salt and pepper to taste
- ½ teaspoon dried tarragon

Directions:

1. Add Brussels, mustard, water, salt and pepper to your Slow Cooker
2. Add dried tarragon
3. Stir well and cover
4. Cook on LOW for 5 hours, making sure to keep cooking until the Brussels are tender
5. Stir well and arrange add Dijon over the Brussels
6. Enjoy!

Nutritional Contents:

- Calories: 83
- Fat: 4g
- Carbohydrates: 11g
- Protein: 4g

Garlic And Cauliflower Mismash

Serving: 4

Prep Time: 5 minutes

Cooking Time: 9 hours

Ingredients:

- 1 large cauliflower head, broken into florets
- 6 garlic cloves, peeled
- 4 tablespoons herbs, minced
- 1 cup vegetable broth
- 4-6 cups water
- 3 tablespoons clarified butter
- Salt to taste

Directions:

1. Peel up the leaves from your cauliflower and cut them up into medium florets

2. Add them to your cooker and top them up with garlic cloves, veggie broth and just enough water to cover the cauliflower

3. Cook on LOW for 6 hours and then on HIGH for 3 hours

4. Drain the water and broth and add the cauliflower back to the cooker

5. Add butter and use immersion blender to mash them

6. Season with some salt and pepper

7. Add herbs for added flavor

8. Serve and enjoy!

Nutritional Contents:

- Calories: 25
- Fat: 5g
- Carbohydrates: 1g
- Protein: 2g

Simple Garlic And Kale Feeding

Serving: 3

Prep Time: 20 minutes

Cooking Time: 5 hours

Ingredients:

- 4 bunch kale, washed, stemmed and cut into large pieces
- 2 onions, chopped
- 8 garlic cloves, minced
- 2 jalapeno peppers, minced
- 4 large red bell peppers, deseeded, sliced
- 1 tablespoon chili powder
- ½ teaspoon salt
- 1/8 teaspoon freshly ground black pepper

Directions:

1. Add kale, onions, jalapeno peppers, garlic, bell pepper to your Slow Cooker
2. Sprinkle chili powder, salt and pepper and stir
3. Cover with lid and cook on LOW for 4-5 hours until the kale is tender
4. Serve and enjoy!

Nutritional Contents:

- Calories: 52
- Fat: 1g
- Carbohydrates: 11g
- Protein: 3g

Keto Friendly Rosemary Flavored Green Beans

Serving: 4

Prep Time: 10 minutes

Cooking Time: 1 hour 30 minutes

Ingredients:

- 1 pound green beans
- 1 tablespoon rosemary, minced
- 1 teaspoon fresh thyme, minced
- 2 tablespoons lemon juice
- 2 tablespoons water

Directions:

1. Add all of the listed ingredients to your pot
2. Cook on LOW for about 3 hours, making sure to stir it from time to time
3. One done, allow it to cool and serve!

Nutritional Contents:

- Calories: 40
- Fat: 0g
- Carbohydrates: 9g
- Protein: 2g

Juicy Summertime Veggies

Serving: 6

Prep Time: 10 minutes

Cooking Time: 3 hours 5 minutes

Ingredients:

- 1 cup grape tomatoes
- 2 cups okra
- 1 cup mushrooms
- 2 cups yellow bell peppers
- 1 and ½ cup red onions
- 2 and ½ cups zucchini
- ½ cup olive oil
- ½ cup balsamic vinegar
- 1 tablespoon fresh thyme, chopped
- 2 tablespoons fresh basil, chopped

Directions:

1. Slice and chop okra, onions, tomatoes, zucchini, mushrooms

2. Add veggies to a large container and mix

3. Take another dish and add oil and vinegar, mix in thyme and basil

4. Toss the veggies into Slow Cooker and pour marinade

5. Stir well

6. Close lid and cook on 3 hours on HIGH, making sure to stir after every hour

Nutritional Contents:

- Calories: 233
- Fat: 18g
- Carbohydrates: 14g
- Protein: 3g

Crazy Caramelized Onion

Serving: 4

Prep Time: 10 minutes

Cooking Time: 9-10 hours

Ingredients:

- 6 onions, sliced
- 2 tablespoons oil
- ½ teaspoon salt

Directions:

1. Add onions, oil and salt to your Slow Cooker.

2. Close lid and cook on LOW for 8 hours.

3. Open lid and keep simmering for 1-2 hours until any excess water has evaporated.

4. Serve and enjoy!

Nutritional Contents:

- Calories: 126
- Fat: 15g
- Carbohydrates: 15g
- Protein: 2g

Broccoli Crunchies

Serving: 4

Prep Time: 10 minutes

Cooking Time: 3 hours

Ingredients:

- 2 cups broccoli florets
- 2 ounces cream of celery soup
- 2 tablespoons cheddar cheese, shredded
- 1 small yellow onion, chopped
- ¼ teaspoon Worcestershire sauce
- Salt and pepper as needed
- ½ tablespoon butter

Directions:

1. Add broccoli, cream, cheese, onion, cheddar to Slow Cooker
2. Stir and season with salt and pepper
3. Place lid and cook on LOW for 3 hours
4. Serve and enjoy!

Nutritional Contents:

- Calories: 162
- Fat: 11g
- Carbohydrates: 11g
- Protein: 5g

The Extremely Slow Cooker Brussels

Serving: 4

Prep Time: 15 minutes

Cooking Time: 4 hours

Ingredients:

- 1 pound Brussels sprouts, bottom trimmed and cut
- 1 tablespoon olive oil
- 1 -1/2 tablespoon Dijon mustard
- ¼ cup water
- Salt and pepper as needed
- ½ teaspoon dried tarragon

Directions:

1. Add Brussels, salt, water, pepper, mustard to Slow Cooker
2. Add dried tarragon and stir
3. Place lid and cook on LOW for 5 hours until the Brussels are tender
4. Stir well and add Dijon over Brussels
5. Stir and enjoy!

Nutritional Contents:

- Calories: 83
- Fat: 4g
- Carbohydrates: 11g
- Protein: 4g

A Green Bean Mixture

Serving: 2

Prep Time: 10 minutes

Cooking Time: 2 hours

Ingredients:

- 4 cups green beans, trimmed
- 2 tablespoons butter, melted
- 1 tablespoon date paste
- Salt and pepper as needed
- ¼ teaspoon coconut aminos

Directions:

1. Add green beans, date paste, pepper, salt, coconut aminos and stir
2. Toss and place lid
3. Cook on LOW for 2 hours
4. Serve and enjoy!

Nutritional Contents:

- Calories: 236
- Fat: 6g
- Carbohydrates: 10g
- Protein: 6g

Roast Peppers with Zucchini

Serving: 2

Prep Time: 15 minutes

Ingredients

- 2 bell peppers, cut in chunks
- 3 zucchini, cut in chunks
- ½ cup garlic cloves, peeled
- Seasoning: salt, pepper, Italian seasoning to taste
- 2 tbsp. olive oil

Directions

1. Add the vegetables and oil to a greased crockpot. Season with salt, pepper and Italian seasoning.
2. Close the lid. Cook for 3 hours on high.

Nutritional Values

- Calories: 97kcal
- Fat: 7.4 g
- Carbohydrates: 7.7g
- Protein: 2.3g
- Dietary Fiber : 7g
- Cholesterol: 24mg

Tomatoes, Asparagus & Squash

Serving: 2

Prep Time: 10 minutes

Ingredients

- 15 oz tomatoes, diced
- 10 oz asparagus, cut in large pieces
- 10 oz summer squash, cut in large pieces
- 10 oz marrow squash, cut in large pieces
- Seasoning: salt, pepper, garlic, onion powder, basil to taste

Directions

1. Add diced tomatoes to the bottom of a crockpot.
2. On top of tomatoes, place the vegetables. Season with salt, pepper and herbs.
3. Close the lid. Cook for 3 hours on high.

Nutritional Values

- Calories: 38 kcal
- Fat: 0.4
- Carbohydrates: 9g
- Protein: 3g
- Dietary Fiber : 3.1g
- Cholesterol: 0mg

Cheesy Cauliflower with Mushrooms

Serving: 2

Prep Time: 10 minutes

Ingredients

- 4 cups frozen cauliflower, thawed
- ½ cup onion, chopped
- 10 oz white mushrooms, sliced
- 2 cups American cheese, shredded
- Salt, pepper to taste

Directions

1. Combine vegetables and mushrooms with cheese in a crockpot. Season with salt and pepper.
2. Close the lid. Cook for 4 hours on low.

Nutritional Values

- Calories: 366 kcal

- Fat: 22g

- Carbohydrates: 18g

- Protein: 25.g

- Dietary Fiber : 2.3g

- Cholesterol: 0mg

Eggplant Parmigiana

Serving: 2

Prep Time: 6 minutes

Ingredients

- 3 medium eggplants, peeled, cut in 2 inch slices
- 1/3 cup seasoned bread crumbs
- ½ cup Parmesan, grated
- 32 oz marinara sauce
- Salt, pepper to taste

Directions

1. Using olive oil, sauté the eggplants in a large skillet until lightly brown.
2. In a separate bowl combine the seasoned bread crumbs with grated Parmesan.
3. Layer the eggplants into a crockpot beginning with eggpland, next top with crumbs, then marinara sauce. Repeat layers.
4. Close the lid and cook for 5 hours on low.

Nutritional Values

- Calories: 353 kcal
- Fat: 13g
- Carbohydrates: 51g
- Protein: 13g
- Dietary Fiber : 3.1g
- Cholesterol: 0mg

Glazed Carrots

Serving: 2

Prep Time: 5 minutes

Ingredients

- 2 lb baby carrots, washed
- 3 tbsp. maple syrup
- 2 tbsp. coconut oil
- ¼ cup water
- Salt, herbs (rosemary, thyme, dill) to taste

Directions

1. Add all ingredients into a crockpot bowl.
2. Close the lid and cook for 5 hours on high. Stir the carrots after 4 hours cooking.

Nutritional Values

- Calories: 70 kcal

- Fat: 1.3g

- Carbohydrates: 14.5g

- Protein: 0.8g

- Dietary Fiber : 3.1g

- Cholesterol: 0mg

Turnip Greens

Serving: 2

Prep Time: 5 minutes

Ingredients

- 3 turnips, peeled, quartered
- 2 bunches fresh turnip greens, washed, chopped
- ½ lb ham hock
- 1 pinch red pepper flakes
- 1 cup water

Directions

1. Add half of greens to a crockpot with 1 cup of water. Add the turnips, ham hock and red pepper.
2. Close the lid and cook for 1 hour on low. Then add the remaining greens.
3. Cook for 6 hours on low.

Nutritional Values

- Calories: 114 kcal
- Fat: 6.7g
- Carbohydrates: 5g
- Protein: 8.6g
- Dietary Fiber : 3.1g
- Cholesterol: 0mg

Bacon-flavored Cabbage

Serving: 2

Prep Time: 5 minutes

Ingredients

- 1 small head of cabbage, cored, chopped
- 2/3 cup cooked, crumbled bacon
- 15 oz pearl onions,
- 8 cups chicken broth
- Salt, pepper to taste

Directions

1. Place the chopped cabbage into a crockpot.
2. Top with onions and bacon. Season with salt and pepper.
3. Pour the broth over the cabbage.
4. Close the lid and cook for 6 hours on high.

Nutritional Values

- Calories: 138 kcal
- Fat: 6g
- Carbohydrates: 11.5g
- Protein: 9g
- Dietary Fiber : 3.1g
- Cholesterol: 0mg

Yellow Squash Casserole

Serving: 2

Prep Time: 5 minutes

Ingredients

- 2 lb yellow squash, sliced across
- 1 cup chopped onion
- 2 cups salted crackers , crumbled
- 1 cup Cheddar cheese, shredded
- 1 tbsp. butter

Directions

1. Microwave squash, onion and 1 tablespoon butter for 10 minutes uncovered.
2. Add the squash mixture together with ½ cup cheese and 1 cup cracker crumbs into a crockpot.
3. In a separate bowl combine the remaining cheese with 1 cup of cracker crumbs, and sprinkle over the squash.
4. Close the lid and cook for 2 hours on low.
5. Turn the heat off and let stand for 30 min

Nutritional Values

- Calories: 97 kcal

- Fat: 5g

- Carbohydrates: 6g

- Protein: 5g

- Dietary Fiber : 3.1g

- Cholesterol: 0mg

Roasted Zucchini with Onion

Serving: 2

Prep Time: 5 minutes

Ingredients

- 2 carrots, peeled, sliced
- ½ onion, sliced
- 2 zucchini, cubed thickly
- 2 tbsp. olive oil
- 1 packet Italian dressing mix, dry

Directions

1. Place the vegetables into a crockpot bowl. Sprinkle with oil and Italian seasoning. Toss well.
2. Close the lid and cook for 6 hours on low.
3. Serve with Parmesan cheese if desired.

Nutritional Values

- Calories: 410 kcal

- Fat: 3.5g

- Carbohydrates: 2.6g

- Protein: 0.3g

- Dietary Fiber : 3.1g

- Cholesterol: 0mg

Chapter 8: Dessert Recipes

The Decisive Dark Chocolate Cake

Serving: 10

Prep Time: 10 minutes

Cooking Time: 3 hours 10 minutes

Ingredients:

* 1 cup + 2 tablespoons almond flour
* 1 and ½ teaspoons baking powder
* ½ cup cocoa powder
* ½ cup granular swerve
* 3 tablespoons unflavored whey powder/egg white protein powder
* ¼ teaspoon salt
* 2/3 cup almond milk, unsweetened
* 3 large whole eggs
* ¾ teaspoon vanilla extract
* 6 tablespoons melted butter
* 1/3 cup chocolate chips, sugar free

Directions:

1. Prepare a six quart slow cooker and grease with oil
2. Add whey protein powder, almond flour, sweetener, baking powder, salt, cocoa powder
3. Fold in butter, eggs, vanilla extract, milk and mix well
4. Stir in chips and pour batter into the pot
5. Place lid and cook 3 hours until a toothpick comes out clean from the center
6. Remove heat and let it cool for 20 minutes, slice and serve
7. Enjoy!

Nutritional Contents:

* Calories: 205
* Fat: 17g
* Carbohydrates: 9g

- Protein: 8g

Heavenly Pumpkin Custard

Serving: 6

Prep Time: 10 minutes

Cooking Time: 2 hours 14 minutes

Ingredients:

- 1 cup pumpkin swerve
- 4 large whole eggs
- ½ cup granulated stevia
- 1/8 teaspoon salt
- 1 teaspoon vanilla extract
- 1 teaspoon pumpkin pie spice
- 4 tablespoons butter
- ½ cup super-fine almond flour

Directions:

1. Grease slow cooker with butter
2. Whisk eggs and blend using a mixer, slowly adding sweetener
3. Blend in vanilla extract and puree
4. Fold in salt, pie spices, almond flour
5. Mix well and add the mixture to Slow Cooker
6. Place lid and place a paper towel between top and fixings to absorb moisture on top of the custard
7. Cook on LOW for 2 -2 and ¾ hours
8. Once the center is set, garnish and enjoy!

Nutritional Contents:

- Calories: 147
- Fat: 12g
- Carbohydrates: 3g
- Protein: 5g

Hearty Slow Cooker Zucchini Bread

Serving: 12

Prep Time: 15 minutes

Cooking Time: 3 hours 15 minutes

Ingredients:

- 1 cup almond flour
- 2 teaspoons cinnamon
- 1/3 cup coconut flour
- ½ teaspoon salt
- ½ teaspoon baking soda
- 1 and ½ teaspoon baking powder
- 1/3 cup soft coconut oil
- 3 whole eggs
- 2 teaspoons vanilla bean extract
- 1 cup sweetener
- 2 cups shredded zucchini
- ½ cup pecans, chopped

Directions:

1. Take a bowl Add coconut and almond flour, salt, baking soda and powder, cinnamon and xanthan gum

2. Keep it on the side

3. Take another bowl and mix oil, vanilla, eggs and sugar, mix well

4. Blend in shredded zucchini and nuts

5. Pour the baking soda into the bowl with zucchini and stir well

6. Pour the mixture into your prepared pan

7. Arrange cooked on top rack and place lid

8. Cook on HIGH for 3 hours

9. Let it cool and wrap in foil, place in fridge

10. Serve and enjoy!

Nutritional Contents:

- Calories: 174
- Fat: 15g
- Carbohydrates: 13g

- Protein: 6g

Simple Cinnamon Cocoa Almonds

Serving: 8

Prep Time: 5 minutes

Cooking Time: 2 hours

Ingredients:

- 3 cups raw almonds
- 3 tablespoons coconut oil, melted
- Kosher salt
- ¼ cup Erythritol
- 1 tablespoon unsweetened cocoa powder
- 1 tablespoon ground cinnamon

Directions:

1. Add almonds coconut oil to the slow cooker and stir until coated
2. Season with salt
3. Mix in Erythritol, cocoa powder, cinnamon and cover
4. Cook on HIGH for 2 hours, making sure to stir every 30 minutes
5. Transfer nuts to a large baking sheet and spread them out to cool
6. Serve and enjoy!

Nutritional Contents:

- Calories: 275
- Fat: 23g
- Carbohydrates: 4g
- Protein: 27g

Delightful Coconut Custard

Serving: 8

Prep Time: 12 minutes

Cooking Time: 5 hours

Ingredients:

- 1 tablespoon coconut oil
- 8 large eggs, lightly beaten
- 4 cups coconut milk
- 1 cup Erythritol
- 2 teaspoons stevia powder
- 1 teaspoon coconut extract

Directions:

1. Coat the inside of your Slow Cooker with coconut oil
2. Stir in eggs, coconut milk, stevia, Erythritol, coconut extract to your Slow Cooker
3. Stir and place lid
4. Cook on LOW for 5 hours
5. Let it cool for 1-2 hours
6. Serve and enjoy!

Nutritional Contents:

- Calories: 375
- Fat: 35g
- Carbohydrates:4g
- Protein: 8g

Chocolate Pot De Crème

Serving: 6

Prep Time: 10 minutes

Cooking Time: 3 hours

Ingredients:

- 6 egg yolks
- 2 cups heavy whipping cream
- ½ cup cocoa powder
- 1 tablespoon pure vanilla extract
- ½ teaspoon stevia
- Whipped coconut cream for garnish
- Shaved dark chocolate for garnish

Directions:

1. Take a medium sized bowl and whisk in yolks, heavy cream, cocoa powder, vanilla, stevia

2. Pour mix into 1 and ½ quart baking dish and place dish in the insert of your Slow Cooker

3. Add just enough water until it reaches halfway up the sides of baking dish

4. Place lid and cook on LOW for 3 hours

5. Remove baking dish and let it cool

6. Chill the dessert completely and garnish with whipped coconut cream and shaved dark chocolate

7. Enjoy!

Nutritional Contents:

- Calories: 198
- Fat: 18g
- Carbohydrates: 3g
- Protein: 5g

Keto Peanut Butter Popsicles

Serving: 2

Prep Time: 15 minutes

Ingredients

- 1 cup peanut butter
- ½ vanilla extract
- 1 cup whipping cream
- ¼ cup granulated sugar
- ¼ cup swerve
- 8 oz. cream cheese
- 4 oz. baking unsweetened chocolate
- 4 pkts Stevia

Directions

1. Mix the peanut butter, vanilla extract, whipping cream, granulated sugar, swerve, cream cheese together.
2. Spoon the mixture into popsicle molds
3. Place a popsicle stick into each mold.
4. Freeze 6 hours or overnight
5. Remove the popsicles by running the mold under hot water.
6. Melt the baking chocolate and add Stevia.
7. Dip the popsicle in the chocolate.
8. Place the dipped popsicles on a parchment paper to cool.
9. Place the dipped popsicles in freezer.
10. Serve it.

Nutritional Values
- Calories: 203kcal
- Fat: 18g
- Carbohydrates: 11g
- Protein: 5g
- Dietary Fiber : 7g
- Cholesterol: 24mg

Yummy Brownies

Serving: 2

Prep Time: 15 minutes

Ingredients

Brownies
- ¾ cup granulated erythritol
- ½ cup coconut flour
- ½ cup butter ghee
- 2 tbsp cocoa powder
- 3 eggs
- 1tsp baking soda
- ½ cup brewed organic coffee
- 6 tbsp. unsweetened almond milk
- 1¼ tsp apple cider vinegar
- 1 tsp vanilla extract

Frosting
- ¼ coconut oil
- 1½ tbsp unsweetened almond milk
- ½ tsp organic vanilla extract
- ½ cup erythritol
- 1 tbsp cocoa powder

Directions

1. Preheat oven at 400F
2. Oil the pan well
3. Mix the coconut flour and erythritol together in a bowl. Set aside.
4. Mix butter ghee with brewed coffee and cocoa powder. Stir and heat to boiling on stove top.
5. Combine both mix and Stir well.
6. Add 3 eggs, almond milk, baking soda, vanilla extract and apple cider vinegar mixture into the combined mixture.
7. Use an electric mixer to mix them together.
8. Pour the mixture into the pan.
9. Bake at 400F for 20 minutes

10. Prepare the frosting by mixing the butter ghee, almond milk and cocoa powder in a saucepan.
11. Stir and heat to a boil. Change to lowest heat.
12. Add erythritol and vanilla extract. Stir well. Maintain lowest heat.
13. Pour warm frosting over the brownies. Use spoon to spread.
14. Cool brownies and frosting.
15. Place it in the fridge for further cooling. Approx. 1 hour.
16. Slice and Serve it.

Nutritional Values
- Calories: 171kcal
- Fat: 16g
- Carbohydrates: 2g
- Protein: 3g
- Dietary Fiber : 2.2g
- Cholesterol: 0 mg

Keto Lemon Curd

Serving: 2

Prep Time: 10 minutes

Ingredients

- 2 organic eggs
- 2 organic egg yolks
- 3tbsp. granulated erythritol
- 6 tbsp. butter cubes
- ½ cup organic lemon juice

Directions

1. Mix the lemon juice, erythritol, egg and egg yolks together in a pan.
2. Add the butter cubes and turn on the stove and adjust to lowest heat
3. Stir well
4. Once the butter melts, turn the heat up to medium-high
5. Stir until thicken.
6. Pour the mix over a sieve or mesh strainer to remove any egg bits.
7. Place it in fridge.

Nutritional Values

- Calories: 200kcal
- Fat: 20g
- Carbohydrates: 1g
- Protein: 3g
- Dietary Fiber : 0g
- Cholesterol: 60mg

Low Carb Cheesecake Brownie

Serving: 2

Prep Time: 30 minutes

Ingredients

Cheesecake Filling
- 2 eggs
- ¼ cup heavy cream
- ½ cup granulated erythritol
- ½ tsp vanilla extract
- 1 lb cream cheese, softened

Brownie
- 2 eggs
- ¼ cup cocoa powder
- pinch sea salt
- ¼ cup chopped walnuts
- ¼ tsp vanilla
- ¾ cup granulated erythritol
- ½ cup butter
- 2 oz. unsweetened chocolate
- ½ cup almond flour

Directions

1. Preheat oven to 325F
2. Butter the sauce pan and wrap the bottom with foil
3. Melt butter and chocolate in the microwave oven in 30 seconds interval until smooth.
4. Mix the sea salt, almond flour and cocoa powder in a small bowl.
5. Beat eggs with erythritol and vanilla until smooth in a bowl.
6. Add the almond flour and beat it
7. Add the butter chocolate mixture and beat it till smooth.
8. Stir well
9. Spread evenly over bottom of prepared pan.
10. Bake 15 to 20 minutes until it is soft in the center.
11. Set aside to cool for 20 minutes
12. For Cheesecake filling, reduce to 300F

13. Beat cream cheese until smooth.
14. Beat eggs with erythritol and vanilla until smooth in a bowl.
15. Pour filling over crust and place the cheesecake on a bake sheet.
16. Bake until edges are set and center is soft. Approx. 35 – 45 minutes.
17. Remove from oven and cool down.
18. Loosen the edge with knife.
19. Cover with plastic wrap and refrigerate for 3 hours.
20. Serve it.

Nutritional Values
- Calories: 381 kcal
- Fat: 34g
- Carbohydrates: 7g
- Protein: 9g
- Dietary Fiber : 2g
- Cholesterol: 156mg

Coconut Oil Candies

Serving: 2

Prep Time: 25 minutes

Ingredients

- 4 tbsp unsweetened cocoa powder
- 1 cup softened cold pressed coconut oil
- 1 tbsp. swerve
- 1 tbsp. vanilla extract
- ½ tsp sea salt
- 3 tbsp. organic unsweetened cocoa powder

Directions

1. Combine the ingredients in a bowl
2. Mix until smooth
3. Drop by tablespoon onto a parchment paper
4. Refrigerate until candies solidify.
5. Store in a covered container in the fridge.

Nutritional Values

- Calories: 76 kcal
- Fat: 8g
- Carbohydrates: 2.45g
- Protein: 1g
- Dietary Fiber : 1g
- Cholesterol: 73mg

Mint Fudge

Serving: 2

Prep Time: 20 minutes

Ingredients

- 2 tbsp. vanilla extract
- 1 tsp peppermint extract
- 1½ cup pumpkin seeds
- ½ cup dried parsley flakes
- 1 cup cold pressed coconut oil
- ¼ tbsp. sea salt
- ½ cup of swerve

Directions

- Melt coconut oil in saucepan.
- Add all ingredients into blender, follow by the warm coconut oil and blend until smooth.
- Pour into a baking pan.
- Freeze it for 4 hours.
- Retrieve and cut into pieces.
- Store in refrigerator to prevent softening.

Nutritional Values

- Calories: 119kcal
- Fat: 9g (66.9%)
- Carbohydrates: 9.5g (19.8%)
- Protein: 4g (13.2%)
- Dietary Fiber : 3.5g
- Cholesterol: 0 mg

Keto Avocado Pudding

Serving: 2

Prep Time: 5 minutes

Ingredients

- 2 avocados
- 1 tbsp. fresh lime juice
- 400ml organic coconut milk
- 2 tsp organic vanilla extract
- 80 drops stevia
- 1 tbsp. Cacao Nibs

Directions

- Peeled, pitted and slice the avocado into pieces
- Add the ingredients into a blender
- Blend until smooth. Sprinkle cacao nibs on top.
- Serve it.

Nutritional Values

- Calories: 292kcal
- Fat: 28.8g
- Carbohydrates: 3.8g
- Protein: 2.7g
- Dietary Fiber : 0g
- Cholesterol: 0mg

Coconut Pudding

Serving: 2

Prep Time: 7 minutes

Ingredients

- 1½ coconut milk
- 1 tbsp. beef gelatin
- 3 egg yolks
- ½ tsp vanilla extract
- 6 tbsp. stevia

Directions

1. Mix the gelatin and 1 tbsp. coconut milk in a small bowl. Set aside.
2. Heat the saucepan and add the remaining coconut milk and stevia.
3. Stir for 3 -5 minutes.
4. Pour the hot coconut milk over the egg yolks and whisk it continuously.
5. Transfer the hot mixture back into a pot and cook for 3 – 4 minutes until thicken.
6. Pour the small bowl of gelatin into the pot and stir well.
7. Pour the mixture evenly into 2 ramekins.
8. Refrigerate it for 3 hours to set it
9. Serve it.

Nutritional Values

- Calories: 291kcal
- Fat: 8.8g
- Carbohydrates: 45g
- Protein: 7.6g
- Dietary Fiber : 1.8g
- Cholesterol: 15mg

Conclusion

I can't express how honored I am to think that you found my book interesting and informative enough to read it all through to the end.

I thank you again for purchasing this book and I hope that you had as much fun reading it as I had writing it.

I bid you farewell and encourage you to move forward with your Keto Journey!

www.ingramcontent.com/pod-product-compliance
Lightning Source LLC
Chambersburg PA
CBHW051310250726
48656CB00004B/1573